Eat to beat

menopause

Eat to beat menopause

Linda Kearns

Thorsons

Thorsons
An Imprint of HarperCollins*Publishers*
77–85 Fulham Palace Road,
Hammersmith, London W6 8JB

The Thorsons website address is: www.thorsons.com

Published by Thorsons 1999
10 9 8 7 6 5 4 3 2 1

A catalogue record for this book
is available from the British Library

ISBN 0 7225 3922 3

Printed and bound in Great Britain by
The Bath Press, Bath

To Maria, Olivia and Jacob

 # Acknowledgements

The creation of this book owes a great deal to Bonnie Estridge, who writes regularly for the *Daily Mail*. The idea of writing a book never really occurred to me until I got to know her, and the extraordinary publicity she provided for me also led to the marketing of the HRT cake by Fosters Bakery. I am also indebted to my young friend Alexa Normandale whose computer expertise was invaluable. Finally, many thanks to my husband, who never lost faith in the original concept of the cake, for his assistance with the book.

Contents

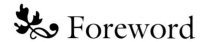 Foreword

It seems that although hormone replacement therapy (HRT) is a wonder-drug for many women who are going through the menopause, there are thousands who just cannot tolerate it as the side-effects are too debilitating. I know that helplines set up to advise menopausal women on alternatives to hormone replacement therapy receive hundreds of calls a week from those desperate to find an alternative.

Two years ago I too decided that I had had enough. I was prescribed HRT at the age of 39 when I had my ovaries removed. I then had an early menopause and although I took various types of HRT for 13 years, it never really suited me. I was always feeling bloated, aching and, on and off, quite depressed. I put up with HRT because it stopped the hot flushes, headaches and palpitations that came with the change of life – but I was not too happy – I've never been one to like taking medicine. However, around that time, I had a real scare ... I discovered a strange dark patch on my breast and I felt sure it was cancer – I'd heard that HRT puts you at risk. In fact, this was not the case, but it scared me sufficiently to ask the doctor whether he thought I should come off HRT. He more or less said 'suit yourself' so I decided to wean myself off slowly and look for other ways to cope. Within a month, the symptoms came back and I made a concerted effort to find a natural oestrogen replacement.

The menopause begins when the ovaries become less responsive to the pituitary gland, the egg-producing cells begin to disappear and oestrogen production falls. It is the reduced level of oestrogen that causes the problems associated with the menopause such as hot flushes, night sweats, lack of concentration and mood swings. Changes in metabolism eventually cause bones to become less dense and may lead to osteoporosis. Increased levels of fats in the blood may lead to narrowing of the arteries and a higher risk of heart disease. To restore oestrogen and counteract symptoms and risk of osteoporosis and heart disease, HRT may be prescribed to replace oestrogen in the body and this is usually given in combination with synthetic progesterone (progestogen), as oestrogen drugs given alone may increase susceptibility to cancer of the uterus. Many women do find HRT of great benefit. However there are also many who are unable to tolerate synthetic oestrogen and wish to find natural alternatives which work for them. It is certainly possible to attack symptoms naturally.

I have always been a wholefood eater and knew that soya and linseed oil are very rich in phytoestrogens – natural chemicals found in plants which mimic female hormones. After coming up with a flapjack-style cake which contained these important ingredients, I tried it myself for a month and found that it certainly seemed to help my menopausal symptoms. I asked around the village for guinea pigs and found ten willing testers who had also – for various reasons – become fed up with taking HRT. All reported back encouraging results – hot flushes, among other things, disappeared within a month. The word got round and I was constantly being asked to bake cakes for friends and friends of friends. Unfortunately, having a full-time job – and a small kitchen! – I just couldn't even attempt to fulfill the demand.

However, being interested in the effect that phytoestrogens appeared to have, I decided to adapt other dishes by including these ingredients and also others that are high in these natural chemicals. A freelance journalist in Leeds called Lesley Hilton had by now heard about my cake and interviewed me for the BBC regional radio. Lesley then contacted Anastasia Stephens, deputy editor of the Good Health section in the *Daily Mail*, who liked the idea and passed it on to journalist Bonnie Estridge. Bonnie interviewed me and one of my guinea pigs. When the article was published, the newspaper was completely swamped with enquiries – literally thousands of women wanted the recipe. The Menopausal Helpline was also completely swamped with letters begging for the recipe. The *Daily Mail* asked me if I would reveal the recipe, and the following week published a colour spread of my 'eat to beat the menopause' recipes including, of course, the cake. The response again was phenomenal. This time, Thorsons approached me about this book and several bakeries expressed interest in marketing the cake. I chose Fosters, a local Yorkshire bakery who set up a special section, Wellfoods Ltd. The Linda Kearns cake Fosters created is faithful to my original recipe and contains nothing but natural ingredients which have not been genetically modified. The response to this cake – which you can now also buy mail-order – has been similarly incredible. John Foster and Janet Woodward of Fosters report orders of tens of thousands – both new customers and repeat orders – every week.

From all the studies I have seen, phytoestrogens (plant oestrogens) appear to be the most effective natural alternative to HRT and are proven considerably to help relieve hot flushes, night sweats, headaches and concentration problems. A study at the Dunn Nutrition Centre in Cambridge showed a significant decrease in menopausal symptoms in women who took 45mg of soya per day (in soya products such as flour, tofu, milk and yogurt). The current estimates of UK intake are known to be as low as 1mg daily. One home-made cake provides seven slices, each of which contains the recommended daily amount of phytoestrogen and the Fosters ready-made cake is similarly calculated, with each cake being enough for 3 days.

There is strong scientific evidence to show that people on a soya-rich diet – for example in China and Japan – have a lower incidence of breast cancer and are also said not to know the meaning of hot flushes. Work in this country also shows that increasing amounts of soya in the diet of pre-menopausal women increases the menstrual cycle by two days. This is thought to be beneficial as it affects the time that breast tissues are exposed to the higher levels of oestrogen produced by the body just before the period begins. In other words, on such a diet over a long time, there would be less exposure to the body's own oestrogen –

 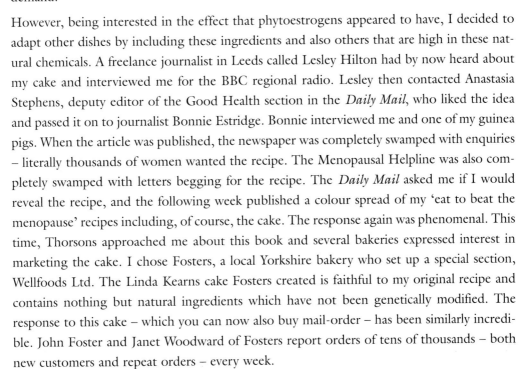

which lowers the risk of breast cancer. We know that phytoestrogens have an oestrogenic effect – but without the possible negative effects that our own bodies' oestrogens produce at certain times of the month. Most foods that are rich in phytoestrogens are familiar (see the list below).

🌿 However, phytoestrogens cannot protect against osteoporosis or coronary disease. My doctor recommended that I take a calcium supplement of at least 500mg daily, which I do faithfully.

🌿 It would also be sensible to look after your heart by choosing vegetable oils such as sunflower, olive or rapeseed oil and eating less saturated fat (dairy products and fatty meats). Use low-fat products and spreads high in poly- or mono-unsaturated fat. Eat at least five pieces of fruit and vegetables a day. Fruit and vegetables contain anti-oxidants – the vital vitamins A, C and E – which help to neutralize unwanted body by-products. They also contain fibre which helps keep the digestive system functioning efficiently, protecting against bowel disease. Supplement a phytoestrogen-rich diet with red-coloured fruit and vegetables: red onions, tomatoes, water melon and pink grapefruit, for instance, contain lycopene which is a type of anti-oxidant that has been shown to help protect against heart disease. Even tomato ketchup contains lycopene in small amounts (but don't over-indulge – it's also high in sugar). Cooking makes the lycopene even more effective – so grilled tomatoes are an ideal food.

Some raw foods containing good amounts of phytoestrogens

🌿 **Cereals**

Oats, barley, rye, brown rice, couscous, bulgur wheat, polenta, buckwheat

🌿 **Seeds**

Sunflower, sesame, pumpkin, poppy, celery, golden linseeds

🌿 **Fruit**

All berries: cranberries, red and blackcurrants, blackberries, raspberries, strawberries, blueberries.

Red grapes (also red grape juice and red wine), currants and raisins

Cherries, plums, pomegranates, all citrus fruit, water melon

Pulses

Soya beans and all soya-based products: soya protein (TVP), soya cheese, soya milk, tofu, soya flour, soya spread (margarine), soya yogurt, soya cream

Chickpeas (garbanzo beans), kidney beans, haricot beans, mung beans, green split peas, broad (fava) beans

Vegetables

Red onions, green beans, celery, sweet peppers (especially red), sage, garlic, parsley root, broccoli, tomatoes, bean-sprouts

Unfortunately, there does seem to be a real backlash against HRT. Maggie Tuttle of the Menopausal Helpline told me that since they set up the service almost four years ago, 9,000 women have contacted them saying that they have tried and simply cannot tolerate it. Some have had particularly adverse side-effects such as breast lumps, confirmed breast cancer, thrombosis, digestive problems, hair loss, joint pains, memory loss, weight gain and severe depression. Sadly, there have also been suicides. We have recently been told that there may be evidence to suggest that HRT could be linked to developing genital abnormalities. Of course, many women take HRT quite happily – but what about the thousands who cannot? Altering your daily diet is an easy and safe alternative.

Menopausal helpline: Send an SAE to 228 Muswell Hill Broadway, London N10 3SH.

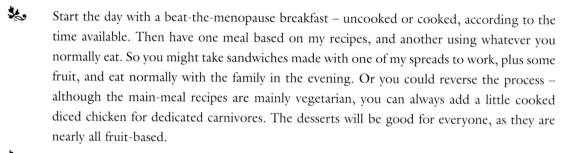

How to use this book

Start the day with a beat-the-menopause breakfast – uncooked or cooked, according to the time available. Then have one meal based on my recipes, and another using whatever you normally eat. So you might take sandwiches made with one of my spreads to work, plus some fruit, and eat normally with the family in the evening. Or you could reverse the process – although the main-meal recipes are mainly vegetarian, you can always add a little cooked diced chicken for dedicated carnivores. The desserts will be good for everyone, as they are nearly all fruit-based.

We all feel the need for a little something to keep us going between meals – make sure yours comes from the book. There are lots of recipes for delicious cakes, cookies and sweet snacks which are quick to make and can be stored in an airtight tin ready for use.

Finally, eat one or more slices of my beat-menopause cake every day. It makes an ideal snack, particularly as it is 95% fat free and has a very good balance of essential vitamins and minerals.

Ingredients

All eggs are large.

Teaspoons and tablespoons are level.

Use either imperial or metric quantities; do not mix the two as they are not exact conversions.

Most recipes containing tofu (bean curd) call for plain fresh, firm tofu; smoked tofu is the same product with a smoky flavour. Silken tofu is softer and more suitable for desserts and making into drinks.

Soya mince (TVP) can be bought ready to use in cans, or in packs in dry form, which needs rehydrating before use.

Breakfast Time

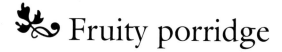 Fruity porridge

Ingredients Serves 2

3oz/75g/1 cup rolled or jumbo oats

1 pint/600ml/2 cups soya milk

1 small eating apple

2 tablespoons raisins

honey and soya milk, optional

Method

 1 Place the oats in a saucepan with the soya milk and bring to the boil. Simmer gently for 5 minutes, stirring frequently to avoid lumps.

 2 Meanwhile prepare the apple and chop it finely. Mix into the porridge along with the raisins. Serve with honey and soya milk if desired.

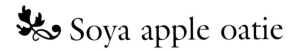# Soya apple oatie

Ingredients Serves 1

1½oz/40g/¼ cup porridge oats

1 tablespoon oat bran

about 300ml/½ pint/1¼ cups soya milk

1 small eating apple

Method

 1 Place the oats, oat bran and soya milk in a small saucepan. Bring slowly to the boil, then simmer for 1 minute. If the mixture becomes too stiff, stir in a little more milk.

 2 Meanwhile prepare and finely chop the apple. Stir into the mixture and serve hot.

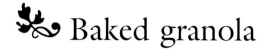 # Baked granola

Ingredients

3 tablespoons sunflower oil

4 tablespoons malt extract

2 tablespoons clear honey

4oz/100g/1¼ cups porridge oats

4oz/100g/1 cup jumbo oats

4oz/100g/1 cup rye flakes

1½oz/40g/6 tablespoons sesame seeds

2oz/50g/⅓ cup pumpkin seeds

2oz/50g/⅓ cup linseeds

4oz/100g/⅔ cup currants

soya yogurt or cream and fresh berries, to serve

Method

 1 Heat the oven to 180°C/350°F/gas mark 4. Place the oil, malt extract and honey in a large saucepan and heat gently until runny.

2 Stir in all the other ingredients and mix thoroughly.
Put the mixture into a large baking tin and bake for about one hour, stirring occasionally to brown it evenly.

3 Leave until cool enough to handle, then break into pieces and store in an airtight tin.

4 Serve with soya yogurt or soya cream and berries of your choice.

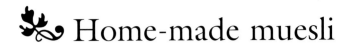 # Home-made muesli

Ingredients

1lb/500g /4 cups jumbo oats

4oz/100g/1 cup oat bran

4oz/100g/1 cup wheat flakes

4oz/100g/¾ cup raisins

4oz/100g/½ cup chopped dried apricots

4oz/100g/¾ cup dried dates

2oz/50g/½ cup dried banana

4oz/100g/1 cup toasted flaked almonds

2oz/50g/½ cup pumpkin seeds

2oz/50g/½ cup sunflower seeds

2oz/50g/½ cup toasted sesame seeds

Method

 1 Put the oats, oat bran and wheat flakes into a large mixing bowl. Add the raisins and apricots.

 2 Chop the dates and bananas into bite-sized pieces and add to the bowl.

 3 Add the pumpkin, sunflower and sesame seeds and mix together thoroughly.

 4 Transfer to an airtight container and store in a cool dry place.

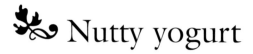 # Nutty yogurt

Ingredients Serves 1

5 oz/150g/⅔ cup soya yogurt

1 tablespoon sesame seeds

1 tablespoon pumpkin seeds

1 eating apple

Method

 1 Put the soya yogurt into a serving bowl and stir in the sesame and pumpkin seeds.

 2 Prepare the apple and chop it finely. Stir into the yogurt mixture.

Variation

Nutty yogurt is equally delicious made with almost any kind of fresh fruit, or with a mixture – for example half an apple mixed with some raspberries.

Toppings, Spreads and Dips

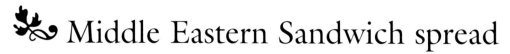 # Middle Eastern Sandwich spread

Ingredients Makes about 1½ lb/700g/3 cups

This is one of my favourite sandwich spreads. It is particularly good on open sandwiches, topped with slices of cucumber and tomato.

½ onion
2 tablespoons sesame oil
½ bunch fresh parsley
1 teaspoon dried basil
½ teaspoon dried oregano
½ teaspoon ground cumin
1½ lb/700g/3 cups cooked chickpeas (garbanzo beans), mashed or blended
juice of 1 lemon
5 tablespoons ground toasted sesame seeds
salt and freshly ground black pepper

Method

 1 Finely chop the onion and sauté in the oil until soft. Meanwhile finely chop the parsley.

 2 Stir in the dried herbs and add the parsley at the last minute, just long enough to soften it.

 3 Put the chickpeas (garbanzo beans) in a bowl with the lemon juice and sesame seeds. Add the onion mixture and stir thoroughly. Season to taste with salt and pepper.

 4 Cover and store in the refrigerator.

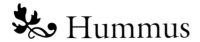 # Hummus

Ingredients

Serve with wholemeal pitta bread or sesame crisp bread, or use as a dip for crudités – fingers of raw carrot and celery.

14oz/400g can chickpeas (garbanzo beans)
1 clove garlic, crushed
1 tablespoon tahini
2 tablespoons sesame oil
2 teaspoons lemon juice
freshly ground black pepper
toasted sesame seeds, to garnish

Method

 1 Drain the chickpeas (garbanzo beans), reserving the liquid. Mash them thoroughly, adding a little of the liquid if necessary to make a workable mixture.

 2 Add the garlic, tahini, oil and lemon juice and mix thoroughly. Add more liquid if necessary – hummus should be creamy but firm. Season generously with pepper and garnish with toasted sesame seeds.

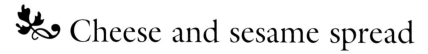 Cheese and sesame spread

Ingredients Serves 4

This nutritious spread is equally good used as a sandwich filler with wholemeal bread, as a toast-topper or for spreading on crispbread.

1 small red onion
5oz/150g/1¼ cups silken tofu
4oz/100g/½ cup cottage cheese
4oz/100g/½ cup soya cheese with chives
2oz/50g/½ cup toasted sesame seeds
1 tablespoon finely chopped fresh chives

Method

 1 Very finely chop the onion. Put the onion in a bowl along with the tofu, cottage cheese, soya cheese and sesame seeds.

 2 Add the chopped fresh chives and stir thoroughly until all the ingredients are combined. Refrigerate until required.

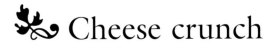 # Cheese crunch

Ingredients

½ celery stick

1 carrot

2 tablespoons natural soya yogurt

2oz/50g/¼ cup soya cheese

1 tablespoon toasted flaked almonds

garlic salt or garlic granules (optional)

Method

   1 Trim the celery, remove any coarse strings and chop it very finely. Trim and grate the carrot.

   2 Put the celery and carrot in a bowl and add the yogurt, cheese and almonds. Mix together thoroughly. Season to taste with garlic salt or garlic granules, if liked.

Sunflower and sesame split pea spread

Ingredients Serves 4

Serve this nutritious nutty spread on crispbread rounds as a starter, or use as a sandwich filling.

8oz/225g/1 cup cooked green split peas
2oz/50g/½ cup sunflower seeds
2oz/50g/½ cup sesame seeds
2 tablespoons soya mayonnaise
salt and freshly ground black pepper

Method

 1 Put the sunflower and sesame seeds in a small frying pan and dry-fry for just a few minutes until lightly browned, stirring frequently. Grind finely in a food processor or with a mortar and pestle.

 2 Mash the split peas, then add the mayonnaise and ground seeds. Stir well to combine with the ingredients and season to taste. Refrigerate until needed.

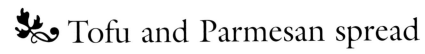 Tofu and Parmesan spread

Ingredients

This spread can be used as a starter or snack, spread on crusty wholemeal bread or sesame crispbreads. Or use it as a filling for jacket potatoes – serves 4.

8oz/225g/1 cup cooked green split peas

4oz/100g/1 cup silken tofu

2 tablespoons soya mayonnaise

2 tablespoons grated Parmesan cheese

¼ teaspoon dried basil

¼ teaspoon dried dill weed

freshly ground black pepper

Method

 1 Mash together the cooked peas and tofu and combine with the other ingredients.

 2 Season to taste with pepper, refrigerate and keep chilled.

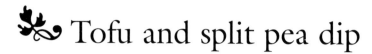 Tofu and split pea dip

This is a very tasty dip, particularly nice with celery sticks, crackers or bread sticks.

8oz/200g/1 cup cooked green split peas
2 tablespoons soya mayonnaise
1lb/500g/5 cups tofu
8oz/225g/2 cups toasted sunflower seeds, ground
¼ teaspoon soy sauce
salt and freshly ground black pepper

Method

   1 Mash the cooked split peas. Add the mayonnaise, tofu and soy sauce. Stir well until all the ingredients are mixed together. Season to taste – you may not need salt as soy sauce is already salty.

   2 Keep refrigerated until ready to use.

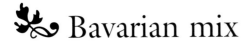 Bavarian mix

Ingredients

Makes enough for 2 sandwiches

2 soya sausages

4oz/100g/1 cup coleslaw

salt and freshly ground black pepper

Method

 1 Cook the soya sausages as directed on the packet. Allow to cool, then slice them thinly.

 2 Stir the sausages into the coleslaw and season to taste with salt and pepper.

Soya cheese spread

Ingredients

This cheese spread is tasty and moist, ideal for use as a sandwich filling or as a toast topper. Alternatively spread it on sesame crispbreads or similar, to make open sandwiches.

4oz/100g/1 cup grated soya cheese
4oz/100g/1 cup grated Edam cheese
½ teaspoon dried dill weed
1 tablespoon soya mayonnaise
freshly ground black pepper

Method

1 Mix the two grated cheeses together. Stir in the dill weed and mayonnaise.

2 Season to taste with pepper (salt should not be needed as the cheeses are already quite salty) and refrigerate until ready to use.

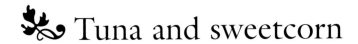 # Tuna and sweetcorn

Ingredients

4oz/100g/¾ cup canned tuna

¼ red pepper

2oz/50g/⅓ cup canned sweetcorn

balsamic or red wine vinegar

salt and freshly ground black pepper

Method

  1 Drain the tuna, transfer to a bowl and mash it roughly with a fork.

2 Core and deseed the pepper and chop it finely. Drain the sweetcorn.

 3 Combine all these ingredients and sprinkle lightly with vinegar. Season to taste.

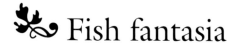 # Fish fantasia

Ingredients

7oz/200g can mackerel in tomato sauce

¼ yellow pepper

½ red eating apple

lemon juice

2 tablespoons soya cream cheese

½ x 7oz/200g can shrimps

salt and freshly ground black pepper

Method

 1 Put the mackerel in a bowl and mash roughly with a fork.

 2 Core and de-seed the pepper and chop finely; add to the bowl.

 3 Chop the apple, sprinkle with lemon juice and add to the bowl.

4 Add the soya cream cheese and mix well. Gently fold in the shrimps and season to taste.

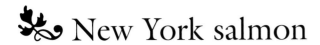 # New York salmon

Ingredients

This classic American sandwich filling is at its best served on fresh rye bread. If you find that too heavy you can buy mixed-grain loaves baked with part rye flour.

4oz/100g/¾ cup canned salmon

2 tablespoons soya cream cheese

½ teaspoon dried dill weed

1 dill pickle

Method

 1 Drain the salmon and mix with the soya cream cheese and dill weed.

 2 Slice the dill pickle thinly and divide between the two sandwiches.

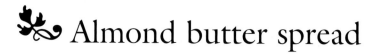 Almond butter spread

An unusual sweet spread, combining creaminess with crunch, this can be eaten on crisp-breads or used as a sandwich filling. Almond butter spread can be found in health food shops.

4oz/100g/½ cup almond butter
2oz/50g/¼ cup soya cream cheese
4oz/100g/¾ cup raisins
2oz/50g/½ cup sunflower seeds

Method

   1 Thoroughly mix together the almond butter and soya cream cheese.

   2 Add the raisins and sunflower seeds and stir well. Keep refrigerated until required.

Tofu and peanut butter spread

Ingredients

This delicious fluffy spread is semi-sweet – use it with the honey in sandwiches, and without as a filling for baked potatoes.

8oz/225g/2 cups tofu
2oz/50g/½ cup raisins or other dried fruit
2oz/50g/½ cup toasted sesame seeds
4oz/100g/½ cup peanut butter
2 tablespoons honey (optional)
salt if needed
chopped spring onions (scallions), to garnish (optional)

Method

 1 Drain the tofu, put in a bowl and mash well. Roughly chop the raisins and add to the bowl.

 2 Stir in the sesame seeds, peanut butter and honey if using; mix together. Taste and add salt if necessary (some peanut butter is already quite salty). Keep refrigerated until needed. If serving on jacket potatoes, garnish with chopped spring onion (scallions).

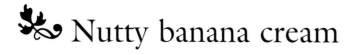 # Nutty banana cream

Although this is a sweet mixture, it is surprisingly successful as a baked potato filling, especially with children.

4oz/100g/1 cup tofu

1 ripe banana

1 tablespoon almond butter

¼ teaspoon nutmeg

Method

  1 Put the tofu in a bowl and mash thoroughly.

2 Mash the banana and add to the bowl together with the almond butter and nutmeg. Use immediately.

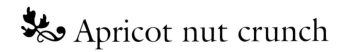 Apricot nut crunch

Ingredients

4 dried apricots

4oz/100g/½ cup cottage cheese

3 tablespoons sunflower seeds

1 tablespoon natural soya yogurt

2 tablespoons finely chopped walnuts

½ teaspoon cinnamon

Method

 1 Chop the dried apricots finely.

 2 Mix all the ingredients together thoroughly. Use immediately or refrigerate until needed.

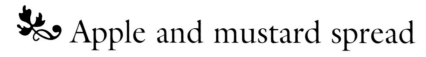 Apple and mustard spread

Ingredients Makes 4 toasts

3 eating apples

10oz/300g/3 cups silken tofu

2 tablespoons soya cream

1 teaspoon wholegrain mustard

salt and freshly ground black pepper

1 tablespoon lemon juice

4 slices wholemeal bread

watercress sprigs or tomato quarters, to garnish

Method

1 Core the eating apples. Grate two into a mixing bowl and combine with the tofu. Add the soya cream and mustard, season to taste and mix well.

2 Heat the grill (broiler). Slice the remaining apple into thin rings and coat with the lemon juice.

3 Toast the bread lightly on both sides. Spread all over with the tofu mixture and grill (broil) for 2–4 minutes until brown and bubbling.

4 Serve hot garnished with apple rings and watercress sprigs or tomato quarters.

Salads

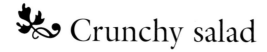 # Crunchy salad

Ingredients

1 bunch watercress

1 red pepper

6 button mushrooms

10oz/300g/1¼ cups bean-sprouts

2 tablespoons soy sauce

Method

 1 Wash the watercress and drain it thoroughly. Discard any tough stalks. Core and de-seed the red pepper, then chop it finely. Wipe and thinly slice the button mushrooms.

 2 Put the bean-sprouts in a salad bowl. Add the prepared vegetables and pour over the soy sauce.

 3 Toss the salad until evenly coated with the soy sauce and serve immediately.

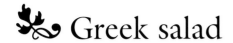 # Greek salad

Ingredients

6oz/175g/1¼ cups hard soya cheese

½ large cucumber

1 red onion

2 large tomatoes

12 black olives

juice of ½ a lemon

freshly ground black pepper

Method

 1 Cut the soya cheese into bite-sized cubes and put into a salad bowl. Dice the cucumber and slice the onion thinly. Finely dice the tomatoes.

 2 Add the vegetables to the salad bowl and mix everything together gently.

 3 Scatter the olives over the salad and sprinkle with the lemon juice. Season with pepper to taste.

 4 Let stand for 20–30 minutes to allow the flavours to develop.

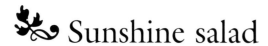 Sunshine salad

Ingredients Serves 2

1 bunch watercress

2 celery sticks

1 small head of broccoli

1 red or yellow pepper

1 carrot

4 tablespoons sunflower seeds

3 tablespoons sesame oil

1 tablespoon balsamic or red wine vinegar

salt and freshly ground black pepper

Method

 1 Wash the watercress and drain it thoroughly; remove any tough stalks. Chop the celery sticks and divide the broccoli into small florets. Core, de-seed and chop the pepper and coarsely grate the carrot.

2 Put all the vegetables into a large salad bowl and stir to mix. Scatter on the sunflower seeds.

3 Mix together the oil and vinegar. Season to taste with salt and pepper and pour over the salad. Mix to coat the vegetables with the dressing. Serve immediately.

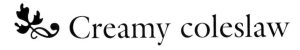 # Creamy coleslaw

Ingredients

¼ red cabbage

¼ white cabbage

1 red onion

2 sticks celery

2 large carrots

8oz/225g/1 cup natural soya yogurt

2 tablespoons pumpkin seeds

Method

 1 Slice the red and white cabbage very thinly using a large sharp knife or a mandolin. Place in a large bowl.

 2 Finely chop the onion and celery and add to the bowl. Grate the carrot over the top.

3 Add the yogurt and stir until the ingredients are thoroughly mixed together. Finish with a sprinkling of pumpkin seeds.

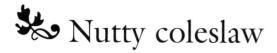 Nutty coleslaw

Ingredients

2–3 tablespoons raisins (preferably the large lexia variety)

4oz/100g/2 cups red cabbage

2 carrots

1 stick celery

2 tablespoons sunflower seeds

1oz/25g/¼ cup chopped hazelnuts

 For the dressing

1 tablespoon Dijon mustard

1 tablespoon olive oil

1 tablespoon lemon juice

½ teaspoon clear honey

salt and freshly ground black pepper

Method

 1 Put the raisins into a heatproof bowl and cover with boiling water. Leave for 10–20 minutes to plump up.

 2 Finely shred the cabbage, coarsely grate the carrots and chop the celery sticks. Pile into a bowl. Drain the raisins and add to the salad.

 3 Pour the dressing ingredients into a screw-top jar, season to taste with salt and pepper and shake to mix. Pour over the salad and toss thoroughly.

4 Sprinkle on the sunflower seeds and chopped hazelnuts just before serving.

Variations

To make a more filling coleslaw, add 3oz/75g/½ cup soya cheese, finely diced and tossed in just before serving.

Four-seed salad with raisins and apricots

Ingredients   Serves 4

1 bunch watercress

1 fennel stick

1 small head Chinese leaves

2oz/50g/½ cup sunflower seeds

2oz/50g/½ cup pumpkin seeds

2oz/50g/½ cup linseeds

2oz/50g/½ cup sesame seeds

2oz/50g/⅔ cup flaked almonds

2 tablespoons raisins

2 tablespoons chopped dried apricots

 For the dressing

3 tablespoons sesame oil

2 tablespoons balsamic vinegar

½ teaspoon clear honey

freshly ground black pepper

Method

1 First prepare the vegetables. Strip the leaves from the watercress and discard the stalks (use in vegetable stock). Chop the fennel and tear the Chinese leaves into small pieces. Put them all into a salad bowl.

2 Add the four seeds, flaked almonds, raisins and apricots to the bowl.

3 Make up the dressing and drizzle over the salad, tossing well.

Marinated tofu with citrus salad

Ingredients Serves 4

8oz/225g/2 cups tofu

2 large oranges

1 bunch watercress

For the dressing

2 cloves garlic, crushed

zest and juice of 1 lemon

2 tablespoons finely chopped fresh parsley

2 tablespoons soy sauce

Method

1 Drain the tofu and cut into bite-sized pieces. Put these in a shallow dish in one layer.

2 Mix the dressing ingredients together in a small bowl. Pour over the tofu cubes and leave to marinate for a good 30 minutes before serving to allow the flavours to penetrate.

3 Meanwhile peel and segment the oranges. Cut the segments in half and put in a serving bowl along with any juice released by cutting. Chop the watercress and stir into the orange segments.

4 Top with the marinated tofu and serve.

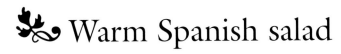 # Warm Spanish salad

Ingredients

8oz/225g/¾ cup brown rice

1 red pepper

4oz/100g/1¼ cups green beans

3 celery sticks

10oz/300g can sweetcorn

7oz/200g can tuna

lemon juice

4 tomatoes

2 tablespoons chopped fresh parsley

2 tablespoons pumpkin seeds

Method

 1 Boil the rice for 20–25 minutes until just tender. Drain and put to one side.

 2 Core, de-seed and chop the pepper. Slice and chop the green beans and celery. Drain the sweetcorn.

 3 Put all the vegetables into a saucepan and pour over barely enough boiling water to cover. Return to the boil and simmer for 3 minutes. Drain well.

 4 Transfer the blanched vegetables to a salad bowl, add the rice and mix together. Drain and flake the tuna, sprinkle with lemon juice to taste and mix with the rice and vegetables.

 5 Quarter the tomatoes and arrange on the salad. Garnish with the parsley and pumpkin seeds.

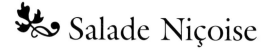 # Salade Niçoise

Ingredients Serves 4

4 eggs

8oz/225g/2½ cups green beans

1 lettuce

1 green pepper

1 red pepper

6 small tomatoes

¼ cucumber, sliced

1 bunch green onions

12 black olives

 ### For the dressing

1 teaspoon Dijon mustard

pinch of sugar

5 tablespoons sesame oil

3 tablespoons lemon juice

1 clove garlic, crushed

salt and freshly ground black pepper

Method

 1 Hard boil the eggs and leave to cool. Cut into quarters.

 2 Trim and slice the beans, then cook in boiling water for just 2 minutes. Drain and leave to cool.

3 Shred the lettuce leaves. Core, deseed and chop the green and red peppers. Slice the tomatoes, cucumber and green onions. Mix them all together in a large salad bowl.

4 Make the dressing by mixing all the ingredients together and seasoning to taste with salt and pepper.

5 Add the beans and olives to the salad and pour the dressing over. Top with the hard-boiled egg quarters.

Variations

This salad comes in many versions, and you can omit or add ingredients according to what is available at the time. Popular additions are drained and chopped tuna or anchovy fillets, and cooked new potatoes, either whole or chopped.

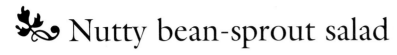 Nutty bean-sprout salad

Ingredients
Serves 4

4oz/100g/½ cup brown rice

2 carrots

4 green onions

1 bunch watercress

4oz/100g/1 packed cup bean-sprouts

2oz/50g/½ cup pumpkin seeds

2oz/50g/½ cup flaked almonds

 For the dressing

2 tablespoons soya cream

2 tablespoons lemon juice

1 tablespoon balsamic or red wine vinegar

1 tablespoon Dijon mustard

1 tablespoon soft brown sugar

4 tablespoons sesame oil

freshly ground black pepper

Method

 1 Boil the rice for 20–25 minutes until just tender. Drain it thoroughly and keep hot.

 2 Mix all the dressing ingredients together, then stir into the hot rice and leave to cool.

 3 Meanwhile prepare the vegetables. Slice the carrots thinly and finely chop the green onions. Divide the watercress into sprigs.

 4 Stir the carrot and onion into the rice and add the bean-sprouts, pumpkin seeds and flaked almonds. Season to taste with pepper.

 5 Spoon the salad on to a serving dish and arrange sprigs of watercress around the edge.

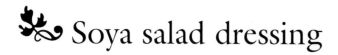 Soya salad dressing

Ingredients

5oz/150g/⅔ cup natural soya yogurt

5fl oz/150ml/⅔ cup buttermilk

1 small green or red pepper

1 teaspoon grated red onion

1 clove garlic, crushed

salt and freshly ground black pepper

Method

   1 Put the soya yogurt and buttermilk into a small bowl and beat together.

   2 Core, de-seed and very finely chop the green or red pepper. Add to the yogurt mixture along with the onion and garlic. Season to taste with salt and pepper. Cover and chill for 30–40 minutes before using. This dressing will keep for up to a week in the refrigerator.

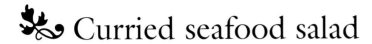# Curried seafood salad

Ingredients

1 small cauliflower
1 green chilli
3 green onions
salt
8fl oz/225g/1 cup mayonnaise
½ teaspoon garam masala
½ teaspoon paprika
1 lb/500g/4 cups cooked peeled prawns (shrimp)
½ lettuce
few fresh coriander (cilantro) leaves (optional)

Method

1 Divide the cauliflower into florets. De-seed and finely chop the chilli; finely chop the green onions.

2 Cook the cauliflower in lightly salted boiling water for 5 minutes, so that it is still quite firm. Leave to cool.

3 Put the mayonnaise in a large bowl with the garam masala, paprika, chilli and green onions. Toss the cauliflower and prawns (shrimp) in the mixture until coated.

4 Serve on a bed of lettuce leaves with coriander (cilantro) leaves sprinkled over the top (optional).

Soups and Starters

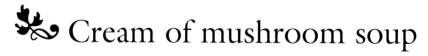 # Cream of mushroom soup

Ingredients Serves 2–3

2 red onions, finely chopped

2 potatoes

8oz/225g/2½ cups button mushrooms

1 tablespoon olive oil

1 clove garlic, crushed

10fl oz/300ml/1¼ cups water

2 teaspoons yeast extract

10fl oz/300ml/1¼ cups soya milk

salt and freshly ground black pepper

Method

1 Finely chop the onions and potatoes and slice the mushrooms thinly.

2 Heat the oil in a large saucepan. Add the onions, potatoes and garlic and stir fry for a few minutes.

3 Add the water and yeast extract. Simmer for 10–15 minutes or until the potatoes are softened.

4 Add the milk and mushrooms and cook for another 5 minutes.

5 Blend or sieve the soup, then return to the pan to reheat. Season to taste.

Celery and green bean soup

Ingredients

2 large red onions

3 celery sticks

4oz/100g/packed cup green beans

1 tablespoon sesame oil

1½ pints/850ml/4 cups water

1 teaspoon yeast extract

pumpkin seeds and chopped fresh chives to garnish

Method

 1 Finely chop the onions and celery and slice the beans.

 2 Heat the oil in a large saucepan and cook the onions for a few minutes until softened but not browned.

 3 Add the celery, beans, water and yeast extract. Bring to the boil, then reduce the heat and simmer for 20 minutes or until the vegetables are tender-crisp.

 4 Serve with a generous garnish of pumpkin seeds and chopped chives.

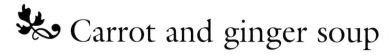 Carrot and ginger soup

Ingredients Serves 2–3

2–3 carrots, washed and sliced

2.5cm/1in piece fresh ginger root

2 red onions

1 pint/600ml/2½ cups vegetable stock (bouillon) (see page 47)

2 tablespoons soya spread

1 teaspoon ground ginger

1 teaspoon grated orange zest

2 tablespoons fresh orange juice

salt and freshly ground pepper

soya cream and finely chopped fresh parsley to garnish

Method

 1 Slice the carrots thinly and finely chop the ginger root and onions.

 2 Put the stock (bouillon) in a saucepan, add the carrots and ginger root and bring to the boil. Partly cover and simmer for about 15 minutes. Remove a tablespoon of carrot slices and set aside for garnishing.

 3 Heat the soya spread in another pan and cook the onions for 3–4 minutes. Then add the ground ginger and cook for a further minute on a low heat.

 4 Add the orange zest and juice, then stir in the carrots and stock (bouillon). Bring to the boil, cover and simmer for 10–12 minutes. Season to taste.

 5 Blend or sieve the soup and return to the pan to reheat. Serve in individual bowls garnished with soya cream, chopped parsley and the reserved carrot slices.

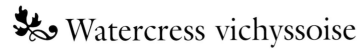# Watercress vichyssoise

Ingredients

1 large red onion

8oz/225g/2 cups leeks

12oz/350g/2½ cups potatoes

2 tablespoons soya spread

1¾ pints/1 litre/4¼ cups vegetable stock (bouillon) (see page 47)

grated zest of ½ lemon

salt and freshly ground black pepper

5fl oz/150ml/⅔ cup soya milk

2 bunches watercress

Method

1 Chop the onion, slice the leeks and dice the potatoes.

2 Heat the soya spread in a large saucepan and stir-fry the onions and leeks for 4–6 minutes.

3 Add the potatoes, stock (bouillon) and lemon zest. Bring to the boil, then cover the pan and simmer gently for 45–50 minutes or until the vegetables are tender. Season to taste.

4 Roughly chop most of the watercress, setting aside a few sprigs for garnishing. Add to the pan and simmer for a further 2 minutes.

5 Blend or sieve the soup, then stir in the soya milk. Refrigerate when cool.

6 Serve chilled, garnished with watercress sprigs.

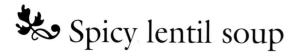 Spicy lentil soup

Ingredients

1 red onion

1 potato, diced

1 carrot, chopped

1 celery stick, chopped

4oz/100g/packed cup green beans

1 tablespoon sesame oil

1 clove garlic, crushed

2 teaspoons mild curry paste

1½ pints/850ml/¼ cups water or vegetable stock (bouillon)

6oz/175g/¾ cup red lentils

salt and freshly ground black pepper

2 tablespoons chopped fresh coriander (cilantro) or parsley to garnish.

Method

 1 Finely chop the onion, potato, carrot, celery and beans.

 2 Heat the oil in a large heavy saucepan. Add the onion and stir-fry for 3–4 minutes, then add the garlic and curry paste and stir-fry for 2 more minutes.

 3 Add the water or stock (bouillon), lentils and remaining prepared vegetables. Bring to the boil, then cover and simmer for 45 minutes or until the vegetables are tender.

 4 Season to taste and serve in individual bowls garnished with coriander (cilantro) or parsley.

Red kidney bean and soya cheese soup

Ingredients

Serves 4

2 tablespoons sesame oil

1 leek

1 clove garlic, crushed

4oz/100g/¾ cup canned red kidney beans

2¼ pints/1.25 litres/5¾ cups vegetable stock (bouillon)

1 tablespoon soft brown sugar

1 teaspoon dried oregano

salt and freshly ground black pepper

2 slices wholemeal bread

olive oil for shallow frying

2oz/50g/½ cup grated soya cheese

Method

 1 Heat the sesame oil in a large saucepan. Slice the leek and stir-fry with the garlic until softened but not browned.

 2 Drain the beans and add to the pan with the stock (bouillon), sugar and oregano. Bring to the boil, cover and simmer for 20–25 minutes. Season to taste.

 3 Meanwhile remove the crusts from the bread and cut the crumb into small cubes. Heat a little olive oil in a small frying pan and sauté the bread cubes for about 2 minutes until nicely crisp. Place on absorbent paper to drain.

 4 Pour the soup into individual bowls and top with the cheese and croutons.

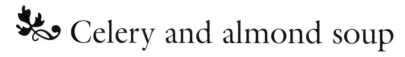 Celery and almond soup

Ingredients   Serves 4

1 head of celery
1½ oz/40g/⅓ cup wholemeal flour
2 pints/1.2 litres/5 cups water
1 teaspoon yeast extract
4oz/100g/½ cup almond butter
salt and freshly ground black pepper
flaked almonds and celery leaves to garnish

Method

 1 Trim the celery, retaining some of the leaves for garnishing. Remove any coarse strings and chop the stalks finely.

 2 Mix the flour with a little of the water in a cup and set aside. Bring the remaining water to the boil in a large saucepan, add the celery and yeast extract, cover and simmer for 15 minutes.

 3 Stir in the almond butter and the flour mixture. Cook over a moderate heat, stirring constantly, until smooth and thickened.

 4 Serve the soup topped with flaked almonds and chopped celery leaves.

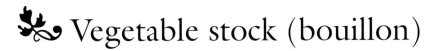 Vegetable stock (bouillon)

Ingredients

Makes about 3 pints/1.75 litres/7¹/₂ cups

Although stock (bouillon) cubes are very convenient to use, they can be rather fatty and salty, and most contain monosodium glutamate and other chemical additives. Vegetable stock is simplicity itself to make at home, and has an excellent flavour as well as being much healthier. Do not season the stock until ready to use. The strained vegetables can be puréed and made into a thick soup.

2 onions

2 carrots

2 potatoes

2 sticks celery

1–2 tablespoons sesame oil or olive oil

3 pints/1.75 litres/7¹/₂ cups water

bouquet garni made up of 1 bay leaf, 1 sprig thyme and 1 sprig parsley (or use a sachet)

Method

 1 Chop all the vegetables roughly (leave the potatoes unpeeled for added flavour).

 2 Heat the oil and add the vegetables. Cook over a very low heat for 5–10 minutes, stirring frequently, until softened but not coloured.

 3 Pour in the water, add the bouquet garni and bring slowly to the boil. Cover and simmer gently for 1 hour or until all the vegetables are well softened. Add a little more water if the liquid reduces significantly during cooking.

 4 Strain and use, or allow to cool completely. Cover and keep in the refrigerator for 3–4 days or in the freezer for up to 3 months.

Variations

Other root vegetables such as parsnip or turnip can be added. Mushroom stalks are also good, but not cabbage or broccoli as they can give an unpleasant smell. If you have a cooked chicken carcass to hand, add it to the ingredients to make your own additive-free chicken stock.

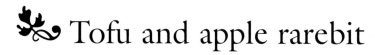 # Tofu and apple rarebit

Ingredients Serves 4

3 eating apples

1 tablespoon lemon juice

10oz/300g/3 cups silken tofu

2 tablespoons soya cream

1 teaspoon whole-grain mustard

salt and freshly ground black pepper

4 slices wholemeal bread

watercress sprigs to garnish

Method

 1 Heat the grill (broiler) to high. Core the apples and grate two of them into a mixing bowl. Slice the remaining apple into four rings and coat with the lemon juice.

2 Combine the grated apple with the tofu. Add the soya cream and mustard, season to taste and mix well.

3 Toast the bread lightly, cover each slice completely with the tofu mixture and grill (broil) for 2–4 minutes until brown and bubbling.

4 Serve garnished with apple rings and watercress sprigs.

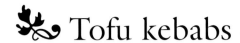 # Tofu kebabs

Ingredients Serves 4

300g/10oz/3 cups tofu

1 red or green pepper

2 red onions

6–8 button mushrooms

wholemeal pitta bread and mixed salad to serve

For the marinade

1in/2.5cm piece fresh ginger root

4 green onions

1–2 tablespoons soy sauce

Method

1 First make the marinade. Finely chop the ginger and green onions and mix with the soy sauce.

2 Cut the tofu into 1 in/2.5cm chunks and put in a shallow dish. Pour over the marinade and leave for at least 4 hours.

3 Remove the tofu and reserve the marinade for basting.

4 Core and de-seed the pepper and cut into even-sized chunks. Cut the onions into similar-sized chunks and slice the mushrooms thickly. Heat the grill (broiler) to high.

5 Arrange the tofu pieces and vegetables in alternate order on skewers. Grill (broil) for 6 minutes, turning once and basting with the marinade, until lightly browned on both sides and cooked through.

6 Serve hot with wholemeal pitta bread and salad.

Soya cream cheese and nut fingers

Ingredients

3–4 thick slices wholemeal bread

8oz/225g/1 cup soya cream cheese (plain or with herbs)

1 tablespoon natural yogurt

4oz/100g/1 cup toasted flaked almonds

Method

 1 Heat the grill (broiler) to high. Cut the bread into 12 fingers and toast them lightly.

 2 Soften the soya cream cheese with the yogurt and spread evenly on the toasted fingers.

 3 Cover the cheese layer with the flaked almonds and firm them down with a palette knife so they stay in place.

Main Courses

Marinated chicken with spicy sauce

Ingredients Serves 4

4 boneless, skinless chicken breasts
sesame oil for frying
fresh coriander and lemon slices to garnish
brown rice with chopped coriander stirred through and mango chutney to serve

 ### For the marinade

3–4 cardamom pods
1 teaspoon coriander seeds
1 teaspoon garam masala
juice of 1 lemon
salt

 ### For the sauce

1in/2.5cm piece fresh ginger root
1 clove garlic
1 green chilli
10fl oz/300ml/1¼ cups natural soya yogurt
1 teaspoon medium curry powder
2 teaspoons paprika
1 bay leaf
1 tablespoon tomato paste
grated zest of 1 lemon

Method

 1 Cut the chicken into bite-sized pieces.

 2 Grind the cardamom and coriander seeds together and combine with the garam masala, lemon juice and a pinch of salt. Spread over the chicken pieces and marinate in the refrigerator for 6–8 hours.

 3 Heat 2–3 tablespoons of oil in a large frying pan. Drain off any surplus marinade from the chicken and cook over a medium heat for 5 minutes until lightly browned and cooked through.

4 Meanwhile prepare the vegetables for the sauce: finely chop the ginger, crush the garlic and de-seed and finely chop the chilli.

5 Remove the chicken pieces to a serving dish with a slotted spoon and keep hot.

6 Put all the sauce ingredients in a small pan and heat gently, stirring constantly. Remove the bay leaf and pour the sauce over the chicken.

7 Serve garnished with coriander and lemon slices, accompanied by brown rice flavoured with chopped fresh coriander and mango chutney.

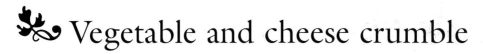 # Vegetable and cheese crumble

Ingredients Serves 4

1½lb/700g/4⅓ cups potatoes

10oz/275g/2 cups young carrots

8oz/225g/2¼ cups green beans

3–4 mint sprigs

1 red pepper

1 bunch chives

3 eggs

15fl oz/425ml/2 cups soya cream

6 tablespoons soya milk

6oz/175g/1¼ cups grated Cheddar cheese

For the topping

6oz/175g/3 cups wholemeal breadcrumbs

2 tablespoons soya spread

2 tablespoons toasted flaked almonds

2 tablespoons sunflower seeds

Method

1 Heat the oven to 200°C/400°F/gas 6. Thinly slice the potatoes; finely chop the carrots and green beans.

2 Cook the potatoes with the mint in a large saucepan of lightly salted water for 8–10 minutes, then add the carrots and beans. Cook for a further 2 minutes, drain thoroughly and put in a large ovenproof dish.

3 Core, de-seed and chop the red pepper and finely chop the chives. Add to the vegetables in the dish.

4 Put the soya cream and milk in a mixing bowl and beat in the eggs and grated cheese. Spoon over the vegetables.

5 Mix the topping ingredients together and sprinkle evenly over the vegetables. Bake for 35 minutes and serve hot.

Cheese and vegetable quiche

Ingredients Serves 4

8oz/225g/2 cups wholemeal flour
salt
4oz/100g/½ cup soya spread

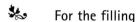 ### For the filling

1 red pepper
1 green pepper
4oz/100g/1¼ cups mushrooms
2oz/50g/½ cup grated soya cheese
8oz/225g/1 cup cottage cheese
5fl oz/150ml/⅔ cup natural soya yogurt

Method

1 Sieve the flour into a mixing bowl with a pinch of salt. Using your fingertips, rub small portions of the soya spread into the flour until the mixture resembles breadcrumbs. Make the dough by adding just enough cold water to produce a rolling consistency.

2 Heat the oven to 220°C/425°F/gas 7. Roll out the pastry and press firmly into an 8in/20cm flan tin (quiche pan). Prick the bottom with a fork. Place on a baking tray and bake empty for 7 minutes or until crisp and brown. Leave to cool. Lower the oven setting to 180°C/350°F/gas 4.

3 Meanwhile prepare the filling: deseed and chop the peppers and slice the mushrooms. Put in a large mixing bowl with the two cheeses and the yogurt; mix thoroughly.

4 Spoon this mixture into the pastry case and smooth the top. Bake in the centre of the oven for 30 minutes or until set.

Variation

Wholemeal pastry has a good flavour but can be rather heavy and difficult to roll out. So if preferred use half wholemeal flour and half white flour to make it lighter.

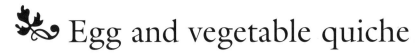 # Egg and vegetable quiche

Ingredients Serves 4

1 pastry case as for Vegetable and cheese quiche

3 eggs

1 green pepper

2 large carrots

2oz/50g/½ cup grated soya cheese

8oz/225g/1 cup cottage cheese

5fl oz/150ml/⅔ cup natural soya yogurt

Method

 1 Make the pastry case, bake empty and leave to cool. Lower the oven setting to 180°C/350°F/gas 4.

 2 Meanwhile prepare the filling: hard boil and chop the eggs. Core, de-seed and chop the green pepper and grate the carrots. Mix with the two cheeses and the yogurt.

 3 Spoon the filling into the pastry case and smooth the surface. Bake in the centre of the oven for 30 minutes or until set.

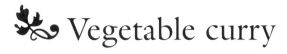 # Vegetable curry

Ingredients Serves 4

4 potatoes
4 carrots
small piece of turnip
1 large red onion
1-2 tablespoons sesame oil
1in/2.5cm piece fresh ginger root
1 green chilli
1 clove garlic, crushed
1 tablespoon ground coriander
1 teaspoon cumin seeds
2 tablespoons tomato paste
1 red pepper
7oz/200g can chickpeas (garbanzo beans)
4oz/100g green beans
1 tablespoon desiccated coconut
salt
1-2 teaspoons lemon juice
brown rice and Indian chutney to serve

Method

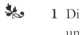

1 Dice the potatoes, carrots and turnip and cook in one pan of boiling water for 5 minutes, until slightly softened but not cooked through. Drain, reserving the liquid.

2 Finely chop the onion. Heat the oil in a large saucepan and cook until softened and starting to brown. Finely chop the ginger root; de-seed and chop the chilli. Add to the pan along with the garlic, coriander and cumin. Cook for a further 2 minutes.

3 Add the tomato paste to the pan with sufficient vegetable water to make a thick gravy. Cover and simmer for about 10 minutes.

4 Meanwhile core and de-seed the red pepper. Drain and rinse the chickpeas (garbanzo beans).

5 Add these to the pan along with the green beans. Sprinkle with the coconut and a little salt, cover and simmer until the vegetables are tender. Season with lemon juice to taste.

6 Serve with brown rice and Indian chutney.

 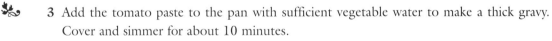

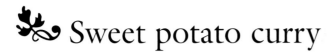 # Sweet potato curry

Ingredients Serves 4

12oz/350g/2 cups sweet potatoes

12oz/350g/3 cups broccoli florets

salt

3 tablespoons sesame oil

½ teaspoon cumin seeds

½ teaspoon fenugreek seeds

½ teaspoon mustard seeds

½ teaspoon fennel seeds

½ teaspoon ground coriander

3 cloves garlic, crushed

2 red onions

1 tablespoon mild curry paste

1 tablespoon tomato paste

brown rice, naan bread or chapatis to serve

Method

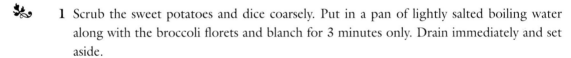 1 Scrub the sweet potatoes and dice coarsely. Put in a pan of lightly salted boiling water along with the broccoli florets and blanch for 3 minutes only. Drain immediately and set aside.

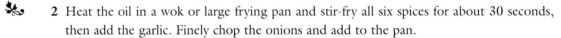 2 Heat the oil in a wok or large frying pan and stir-fry all six spices for about 30 seconds, then add the garlic. Finely chop the onions and add to the pan.

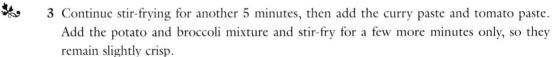 3 Continue stir-frying for another 5 minutes, then add the curry paste and tomato paste. Add the potato and broccoli mixture and stir-fry for a few more minutes only, so they remain slightly crisp.

4 Serve with brown rice, naan bread or chapatis.

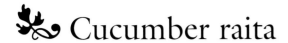 # Cucumber raita

Ingredients Serves 4

1 cucumber
salt and freshly ground black pepper
10fl oz/300ml/²⁄₃ cup natural soya yogurt
2 tablespoons finely chopped fresh mint
1 tablespoon finely chopped fresh chives

Method

1 Thinly slice the cucumber, place in a sieve and sprinkle with salt. Leave to drain for about 30 minutes.

2 Meanwhile put the yogurt in a serving dish with half of the mint and all the chives.

3 Pat the cucumber slices dry on absorbent paper and add to the serving dish. Season generously with pepper and stir well. Chill until needed.

4 Garnish with the remaining mint and serve as a cooling accompaniment to a curry.

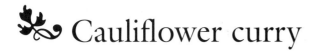 # Cauliflower curry

Ingredients   Serves 3–4

1 red onion

1 small cauliflower

1 aubergine (eggplant)

1 large potato

salt

2 tablespoons sesame oil

½ teaspoon mustard seeds

½ teaspoon cumin seeds

½ teaspoon turmeric

1 teaspoon garam masala

4oz/100g/1 cup peas, thawed if frozen

1 tomato

juice of ½ lemon

brown rice to serve

Method

1 Finely chop the onion, divide the cauliflower into florets, dice the aubergine (eggplant) and cut the potato into bite-sized chunks.

2 Put the potato in a pan of lightly salted boiling water and cook for a few minutes only, until softened but not cooked through. Drain immediately, reserving the liquid.

3 Heat the oil in a large heavy pan which has a lid. Add the onion and mustard seeds, cover and cook until the seeds stop popping and the lid can be removed. Add the cumin seeds and cook gently for a few minutes, then stir in the cauliflower, aubergine (eggplant) and potato.

4 Add enough of the reserved water to simmer the vegetables and sprinkle on the turmeric and ½ teaspoon of salt. Cover and cook over a low heat until the vegetables are softening, stirring occasionally.

5 Sprinkle in the garam masala, add the peas and cook for a further 5 minutes. Chop the tomato and add at the last minute. Finish with the lemon juice and serve with brown rice.

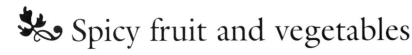 # Spicy fruit and vegetables

Ingredients   Serves 4–6

1 red onion

4 celery sticks

1 tablespoon sesame oil

1 tablespoon garam masala

1 tablespoon wholemeal flour

1in/2.5cm piece fresh ginger root

10fl oz/300ml/1¼ cups vegetable stock (bouillon) or water

grated zest and juice of 1 lemon

1lb/500 g/4 cups cooking apples

2 green, or unripe bananas

4oz/100g/scant cup raisins

8-10 dried apricots, soaked overnight

5fl oz/150ml/⅔ cup soya cream

lemon wedges and fresh coriander to garnish

brown rice, naan bread or chapatis to serve

Method

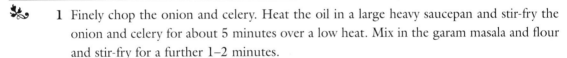 1 Finely chop the onion and celery. Heat the oil in a large heavy saucepan and stir-fry the onion and celery for about 5 minutes over a low heat. Mix in the garam masala and flour and stir-fry for a further 1–2 minutes.

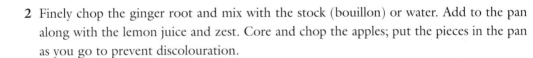 2 Finely chop the ginger root and mix with the stock (bouillon) or water. Add to the pan along with the lemon juice and zest. Core and chop the apples; put the pieces in the pan as you go to prevent discolouration.

3 Slice the bananas thickly and add to the pan along with the raisins and drained apricots.

4 Cover the pan and cook over a low heat for 10 minutes or until the apple pieces are tender.

5 Stir in the soya cream, garnish with lemon wedges and fresh coriander and serve with brown rice, naan bread or chapatis.

Nutty brown rice

Brown rice is much better for you than white as it is unpolished and still has a layer of bran, which gives a nutty flavour and chewy texture as well as the brown colour. The long cooking times of 40–45 minutes recommended in old cookbooks are not necessary – provided you start it in boiling water and not cold, 20 minutes should be sufficient.

Ingredients   Serves 4

1 tablespoon sesame oil

8oz/225g/1 packed cup brown rice

1 pint/600ml/2½ cups boiling water

1–2 teaspoons yeast extract

4oz/100g/scant cup raisins

4oz/100g/1 cup sunflower seeds

4oz/100g/1 cup flaked almonds

Method

   1 Heat the oil in a large pan. Add the rice and toss in the oil for about 1 minute until it becomes translucent.

   2 Add the water, bring back to the boil, then stir in the yeast extract. Turn the heat as low as possible, cover the pan and leave the rice to cook for 20 minutes, without lifting the lid or stirring.

    3 The rice should be almost tender and the liquid nearly absorbed. Gently stir in the raisins, sunflower seeds and almonds and heat for a few more minutes.

Pasta with almond butter sauce

Ingredients

8oz/225g dried pasta

salt

2 tablespoons chopped fresh parsley and basil

2oz/50g/¼ cup almond butter

1oz/25g/¼ cup wholemeal flour

15fl oz/425ml/2 cups soya milk

yeast extract

cayenne pepper

chopped fresh parsley and sliced tomato to garnish

broccoli to serve

Method

 1 Cook the pasta in lightly salted boiling water until soft but still firm to the bite. Drain and toss in the chopped herbs.

 2 Meanwhile make the sauce. Put the almond butter in a pan and gradually stir in the flour. Cook for a few minutes, stirring constantly. Gradually add the soya milk, bring to the boil, then simmer, stirring constantly, until thickened. Flavour with yeast extract to taste and a pinch of cayenne pepper.

 3 Put the pasta in a heated serving bowl or individual dishes. Pour over the sauce and garnish with parsley and tomato. Serve with broccoli.

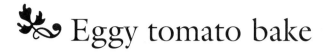 # Eggy tomato bake

Ingredients   Serves 4

8oz/225g/1¼ cups tomatoes

8oz/225g/1 cup courgettes (zucchini)

2oz/50g/¼ cup almond butter

2 onions

1 green or yellow pepper

5fl oz/150ml/⅔ cup dry white wine

2 teaspoons chopped mixed dried herbs

4 tomatoes

4 hard-boiled eggs

2oz/50g/1 cup fresh wholemeal breadcrumbs

2oz/50g/½ cup grated soya cheese

broccoli and carrots to serve

Method

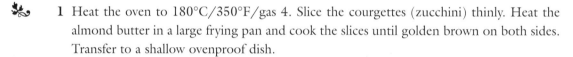 1 Heat the oven to 180°C/350°F/gas 4. Slice the courgettes (zucchini) thinly. Heat the almond butter in a large frying pan and cook the slices until golden brown on both sides. Transfer to a shallow ovenproof dish.

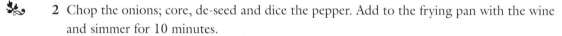 2 Chop the onions; core, de-seed and dice the pepper. Add to the frying pan with the wine and simmer for 10 minutes.

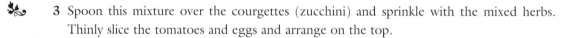 3 Spoon this mixture over the courgettes (zucchini) and sprinkle with the mixed herbs. Thinly slice the tomatoes and eggs and arrange on the top.

4 Cover with breadcrumbs and grated cheese and bake in the centre of the oven for 30 minutes or until golden brown. Serve with broccoli and carrots.

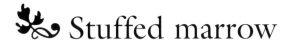 Stuffed marrow

Ingredients   Serves 4

4oz/100g/1 packed ½ cup brown rice

10fl oz/300ml/1¼ cups boiling water

2 onions

1 red pepper

4 hard-boiled eggs

1–2 teaspoons yeast extract

1 teaspoon grated fresh horseradish or 1 tablespoon horseradish cream

celery salt

1 medium marrow

2oz/50g/½ cup tahini (ground sesame seeds, available from whole food shops)

2oz/50g/1 cup fresh wholemeal breadcrumbs

Method

1 Put the rice in a pan, pour in the boiling water and stir briskly. Cover the pan and turn the heat as low as possible. Simmer for 15–20 minutes or until all the liquid has been absorbed.

2 Meanwhile chop the onions finely; core, de-seed and dice the pepper and chop the eggs. Heat the oven to 190°C/375°F/gas 5.

3 Stir the yeast extract into the rice and add the onions, pepper, eggs and horseradish. Season to taste with celery salt.

4 Halve the marrow lengthways and scoop out the seeds. Pack each half with the rice stuffing.

5 Grease an ovenproof dish with half the tahini and put in the stuffed marrow halves. Top them with the crumbs and remaining tahini. Bake in the centre of the oven for 35–40 minutes.

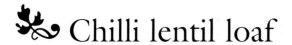 Chilli lentil loaf

Ingredients Serves 4

6oz/175g/scant cup green lentils

1 onion

1 green chilli

1 tablespoon sesame oil

4oz/100g/2 cups fresh wholemeal breadcrumbs

2 tablespoons chopped fresh parsley

1 tablespoon soy sauce

salt and freshly ground black pepper

4 tablespoons dried breadcrumbs, to coat

For the dressing

4 tablespoons natural soya yogurt

1 tablespoon very finely chopped chives

Method

1 Boil the lentils in a saucepan containing three times their volume in water, for 45 minutes or until tender. Drain well and mash.

2 Meanwhile chop the onion; de-seed and chop the chilli. Heat the oil in a large frying pan and cook the onion over a low heat for 5–6 minutes, then add the chilli and cook for a further 2 minutes.

3 Heat the oven to 180°C/350°F/gas 4, and lightly oil a baking tin.

4 Stir the onion and chilli mixture into the mashed lentils. Add the fresh breadcrumbs, parsley and soy sauce. Mix thoroughly and season to taste with salt and pepper.

5 Turn out on to a work surface and form into a loaf shape. Coat with the dried breadcrumbs and lift into the prepared tin with a fish slice. Bake for 30–40 minutes until golden brown and crisp on top.

6 Mix the dressing ingredients together, season with salt and pepper and serve in a small dish.

Soya cannelloni with olives

Ingredients   Serves 3

6 cannelloni (large pasta tubes)

15g/425g can soya mince

1 teaspoon chopped fresh thyme or parsley

1 teaspoon sugar

1 tablespoon tomato paste

8 stuffed green olives

3–4 tablespoons grated soya cheese

tomato slices and chopped parsley to garnish

For the cheese sauce

2 tablespoons soya spread

2 tablespoons flour

10fl oz/300ml/1¼ cups soya milk

4oz/100g/1 cup grated soya cheese

Method

1 First make the cheese sauce. Heat the soya spread in a small saucepan, stir in the flour and cook over a low heat for a few minutes. Gradually add the soya milk, bring to the boil, then simmer, stirring constantly, until thickened. Stir in the grated cheese and remove from the heat.

2 Heat the oven to 180°C/350°F/gas 4. Cook the pasta tubes in lightly salted boiling water for 10 minutes or until just tender. Drain and leave to cool.

3 Put the soya mince, herbs, sugar and tomato paste in a bowl. Slice the olives into the mixture, reserving a few for garnishing.

4 Using a teaspoon, fill the pasta tubes. Place in a shallow ovenproof dish, pour the cheese sauce over and sprinkle with grated soya cheese.

5 Bake in the centre of the oven for 20 minutes until golden and bubbling. Serve garnished with sliced tomatoes, parsley and the reserved olives.

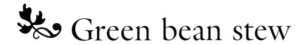 # Green bean stew

Ingredients Serves 4

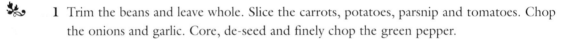

1lb/500g green beans

2 small carrots

2 potatoes

1 small parsnip

1lb/500g/tomatoes

2 onions

2 cloves garlic

1 green pepper

2 tablespoons sunflower oil

1 tablespoon chopped fresh chervil, savory or sage

½ teaspoon yeast extract

Method

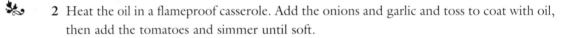

1 Trim the beans and leave whole. Slice the carrots, potatoes, parsnip and tomatoes. Chop the onions and garlic. Core, de-seed and finely chop the green pepper.

2 Heat the oil in a flameproof casserole. Add the onions and garlic and toss to coat with oil, then add the tomatoes and simmer until soft.

3 Add the beans, carrots, potatoes and parsnip. Cover and simmer gently for 30 minutes, until all the vegetables are soft.

4 Finally add the chopped green pepper; simmer for a further 5 minutes, then add the chopped herbs and yeast extract. Serve with crusty wholemeal bread.

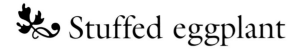 # Stuffed eggplant

Ingredients Serves 4

4 aubergines (eggplants)

1 large onion

2 carrots

½in/1cm piece fresh ginger root

2oz/50g/¼ cup soya spread

4oz/100g/1 cup peas, thawed if frozen

7oz/200g/1 cup canned chopped tomatoes

½ teaspoon paprika

salt and freshly ground black pepper

2 tablespoons toasted flaked almonds

fresh parsley to garnish

brown rice and Cucumber raita (page 59) to serve

Method

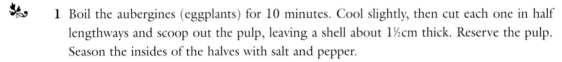

1 Boil the aubergines (eggplants) for 10 minutes. Cool slightly, then cut each one in half lengthways and scoop out the pulp, leaving a shell about 1½cm thick. Reserve the pulp. Season the insides of the halves with salt and pepper.

2 Chop the onion, dice the carrots and finely chop the root ginger. Heat the soya spread in a large saucepan and fry the ginger and onion until softened but not browned. Add the carrots and peas. Heat the oven to 180°C/350°F/gas 4.

3 Chop the reserved pulp and add to the pan with the tomatoes. Cover and simmer for 15–20 minutes until all the vegetables are just tender, adding a little water if the mixture gets too dry.

4 Stir in the paprika and season to taste. Place the prepared halves in a baking tin and fill with the vegetable mixture. Cook for about 20 minutes until golden brown.

5 Sprinkle with the almonds, garnish with fresh parsley and serve with brown rice and Cucumber raita.

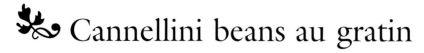 # Cannellini beans au gratin

Ingredients Serves 4

1 large onion

2 tablespoons sesame oil

1 clove garlic, crushed

2 x 14oz/400g cans cannellini beans

salt and freshly ground black pepper

4oz/100g/2 cups fresh wholemeal breadcrumbs

2 tablespoons chopped fresh parsley or savory

broccoli and tomatoes to serve

Method

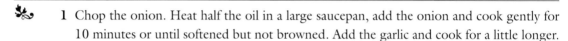 1 Chop the onion. Heat half the oil in a large saucepan, add the onion and cook gently for 10 minutes or until softened but not browned. Add the garlic and cook for a little longer.

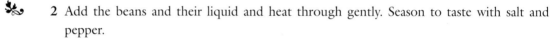 2 Add the beans and their liquid and heat through gently. Season to taste with salt and pepper.

3 Pour the mixture into a shallow ovenproof dish. Mix the breadcrumbs with the herbs and remaining oil, rubbing the oil in lightly with your fingertips to distribute it.

4 Sprinkle the topping mixture evenly over the beans and place under a moderate grill (broiler) for a few minutes until heated through and golden brown on top. Serve with broccoli and grilled (broiled) tomatoes.

Vegetable, seed and oatflake loaf

Ingredients

3 tablespoons sesame oil

4oz/100g/1 cup chopped onion

1lb/500g/5 cups oatflakes (rolled oats)

1½lb/700g courgettes (zucchini)

4oz/100g/1 cup grated Edam cheese

2 eggs

4oz/100g/1 cup wheatgerm

4oz/100g1 cup toasted sunflower seeds

¼ teaspoon nutmeg

salt and freshly ground black pepper

Method

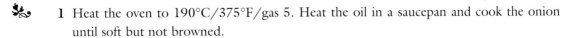 1 Heat the oven to 190°C/375°F/gas 5. Heat the oil in a saucepan and cook the onion until soft but not browned.

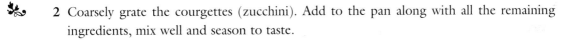 2 Coarsely grate the courgettes (zucchini). Add to the pan along with all the remaining ingredients, mix well and season to taste.

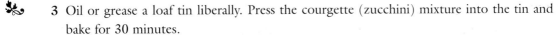 3 Oil or grease a loaf tin liberally. Press the courgette (zucchini) mixture into the tin and bake for 30 minutes.

Lentil purée

Ingredients

1 onion

1 green chilli

1in/2.5cm piece fresh ginger root

8oz/225g/scant cup red lentils

1 bay leaf

1 teaspoon turmeric

2 teaspoons ground coriander

2 teaspoons ground cumin

salt and freshly ground black pepper

Method

 1 Chop the onion, de-seed and chop the chilli and grate the ginger root.

 2 Put the lentils into a large saucepan with the prepared vegetables. Add the bay leaf, turmeric and enough cold water to cover. Bring to the boil, then cover and simmer over a very low heat for 25 minutes or until the lentils and onion are tender.

3 Remove from the heat and stir in the cumin and coriander. Cover and leave to stand for 30 minutes, to allow the flavours to develop. Reheat gently, stirring well until the mixture is creamy. Season to taste.

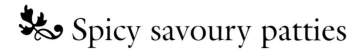 # Spicy savoury patties

Ingredients Makes 24

½ red onion

1 celery stick

½ green pepper

2 tablespoons sesame oil

20oz/600g/6 cups tofu

1 egg

2 tablespoons wholemeal flour

½ teaspoon salt

2 tablespoons soy sauce

1 teaspoon ground coriander

1 teaspoon ground cumin

½ teaspoon paprika

sesame seeds for coating

Method

 1 Finely chop the onion and celery. Core, de-seed and finely chop the pepper.

 2 Heat the oil in a large frying pan and cook the prepared vegetables over a low heat for 5–10 minutes until softened but not browned.

 3 Strain off the moisture from the tofu, put in a mixing bowl and mash. Lightly beat the egg and stir into the bowl along with the flour, salt and soy sauce. Finally add the vegetables and spices; mix well.

 4 Shape the mixture into small patties and roll in sesame seeds until coated. Cook on a preheated griddle or non-stick frying pan for a few minutes, turning once, until lightly browned.

Variation

If more convenient the patties can be baked in the oven at 180°C/350°F/gas 4 for about 20 minutes.

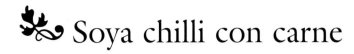 Soya chilli con carne

Ingredients Serves 4–6

1lb/500g soya mince

2 red onions

1 green chilli

2 tablespoons sesame oil

14oz/400g can chopped tomatoes

2 x14oz/400g cans red kidney beans

1 teaspoon crushed cumin seeds or ground cumin

salt and freshly ground black pepper

Method

1 Re-hydrate the soya mince according to the packet instructions. Drain well. Finely chop the onions; de-seed and finely chop the chilli.

2 Heat the oil in a large heavy-based saucepan over a low heat and cook the onions until soft but not browned.

3 Stir in the soya mince and continue stir-frying until it browns. Stir in the tomatoes, drained kidney beans and the prepared chilli. Sprinkle with the cumin and season to taste.

4 Cover and cook over a very low heat for 30 minutes. Stir occasionally and if necessary add a little water.

5 Serve English style with wholemeal bread or brown rice and a green salad; or Mexican style with tortilla chips, sprinkled with cumin seeds and chilli powder and accompanied by tomato salsa.

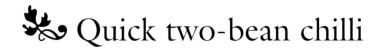 # Quick two-bean chilli

Ingredients

2 red onions

2 carrots

1 red, 1 yellow and 1 green pepper

2 celery sticks

4oz/100g/1 packed cup green beans

8oz/225g can soya beans

8oz/225g can red kidney beans

2 tablespoons olive oil

14oz/400g can chopped tomatoes

1 small jar passata (strained crushed tomatoes) or 1 can condensed tomato soup

2–4 teaspoons chilli powder

sweet potatoes, jacket potatoes or brown rice to serve

Method

 1 Finely chop the onions and carrots. Core, de-seed and slice the peppers. Chop the celery and slice the green beans. Drain the canned beans.

 2 Heat the oil in a large saucepan, add the onions and cook gently until soft.

 3 Add the remaining vegetables and the drained beans; cook for 5 minutes. Pour in the chopped tomatoes and passata or soup and season with chilli powder to taste.

 4 Mix thoroughly and simmer for 10 minutes. Serve with potatoes or rice.

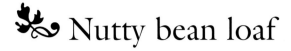 Nutty bean loaf

Ingredients Serves 4

1 small red onion

2 tablespoons olive oil

14oz/400g can chickpeas (garbanzo beans) or soya beans, drained

4oz/100g/2 cups fresh wholemeal breadcrumbs

2oz/50g/½ cup sunflower seeds

2oz/50g/½ cup pumpkin seeds

1 tablespoon tomato paste or ketchup

2 tablespoons yeast extract

2 tablespoons soya flour

2 eggs, lightly beaten

125ml/4fl oz/½ cup vegetable stock (bouillon)

1 tablespoon sesame seeds

broccoli or green salad to serve

Method

 1 Heat the oven to 190°C/375°F/gas 5 and grease a small loaf tin.

 2 Finely chop the onion. Heat the oil in a saucepan and fry the onion for a few minutes to soften. Add all the remaining ingredients except the sesame seeds.

 3 Pour the mixture into the prepared tin and cover with foil. Bake for 30 minutes or until firm.

 4 Remove the foil, sprinkle with sesame seeds and bake for a further 10 minutes. Serve with broccoli or green salad.

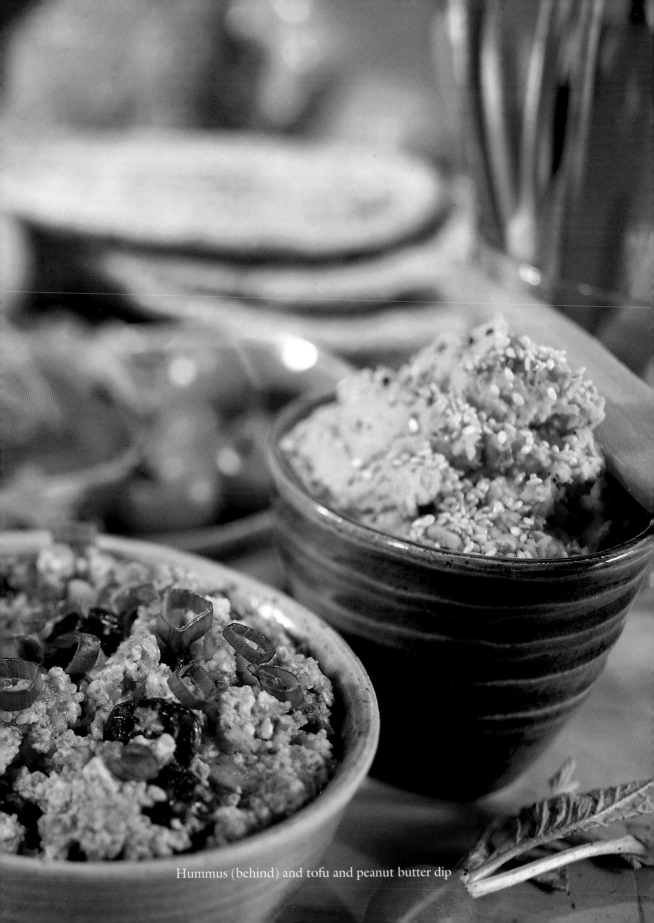

Hummus (behind) and tofu and peanut butter dip

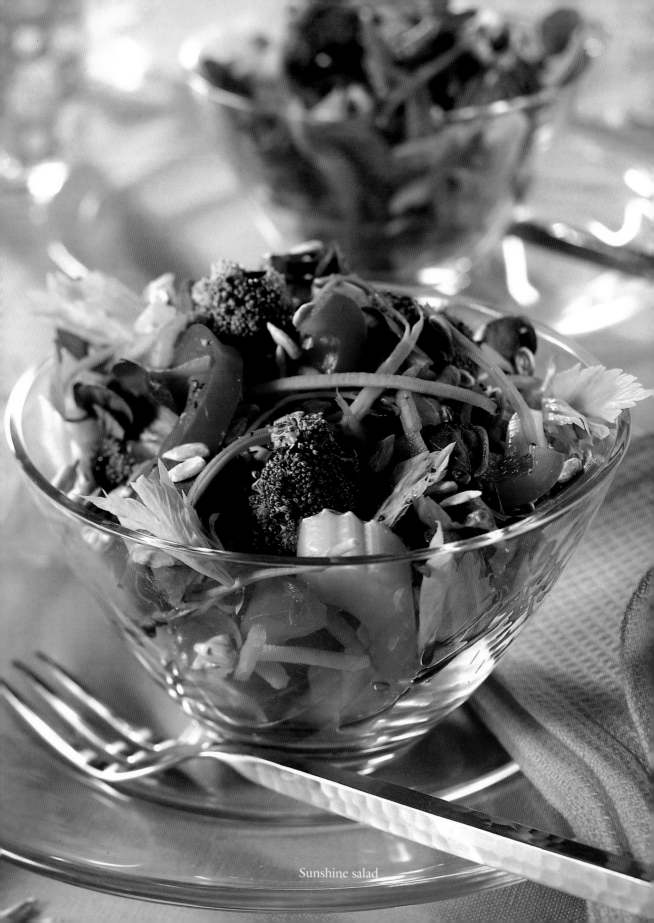

Sunshine salad

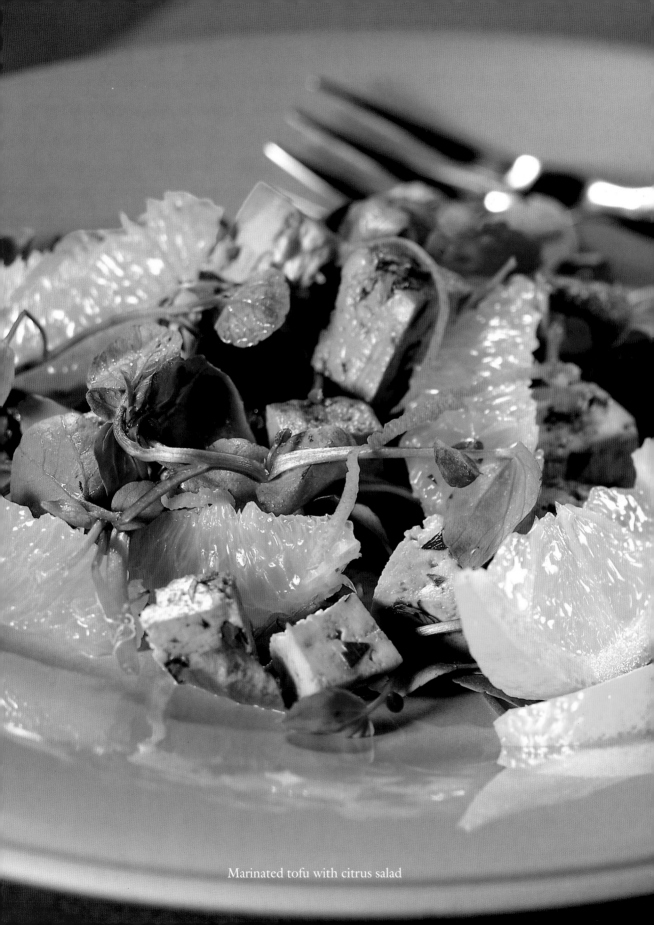

Marinated tofu with citrus salad

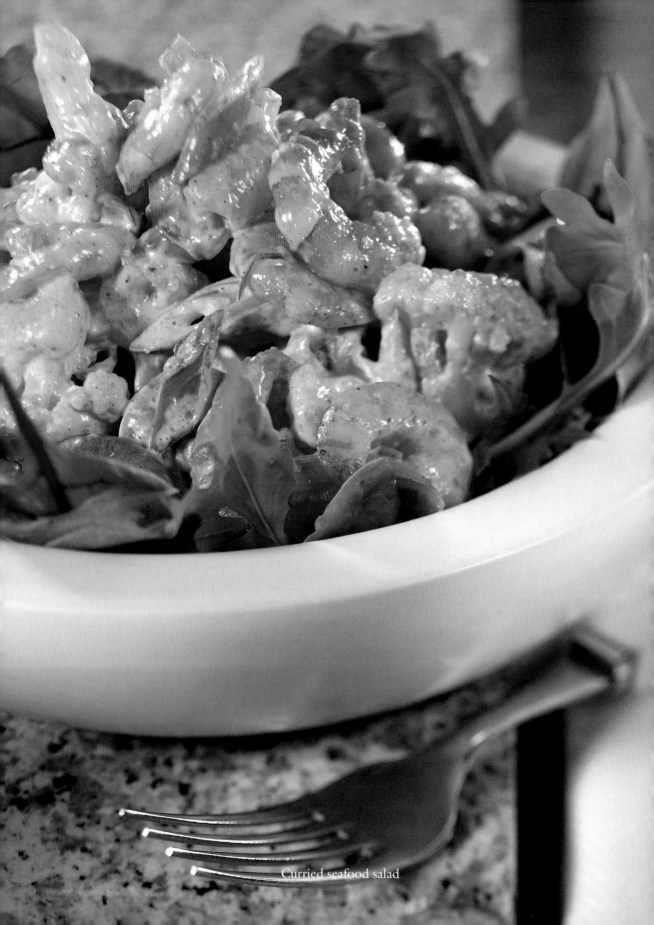

Curried seafood salad

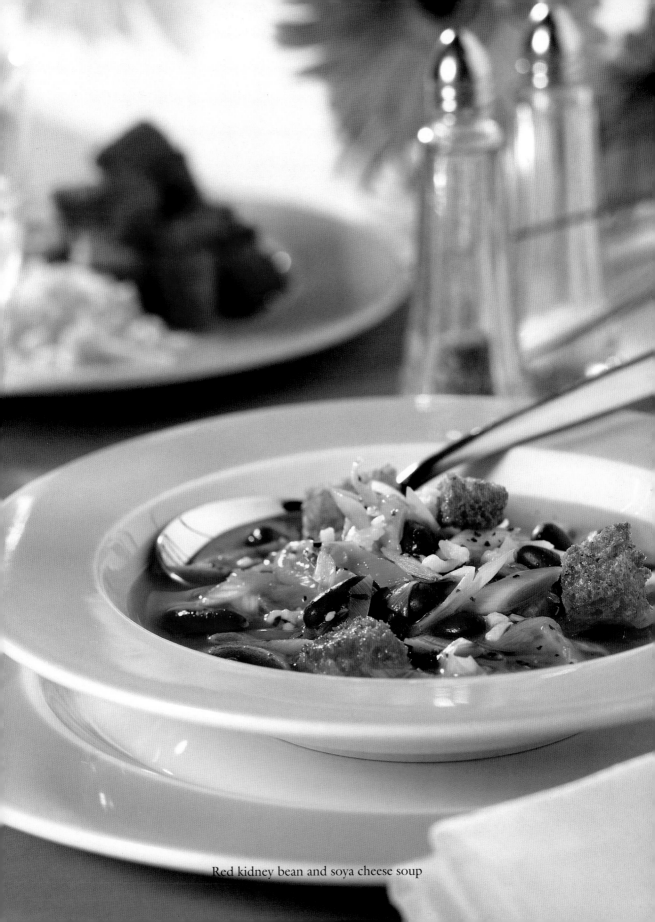

Red kidney bean and soya cheese soup

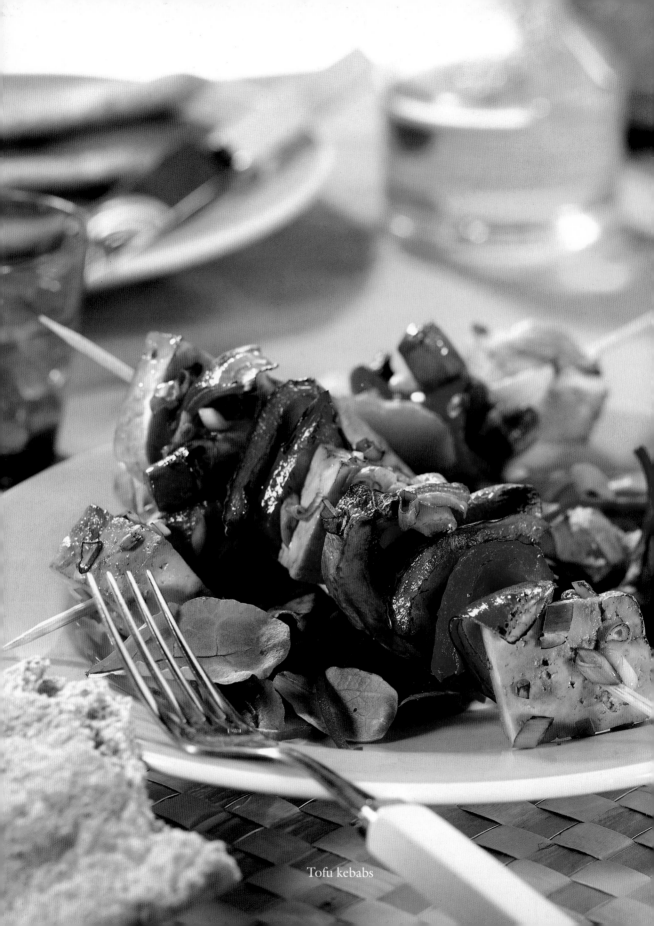

Tofu kebabs

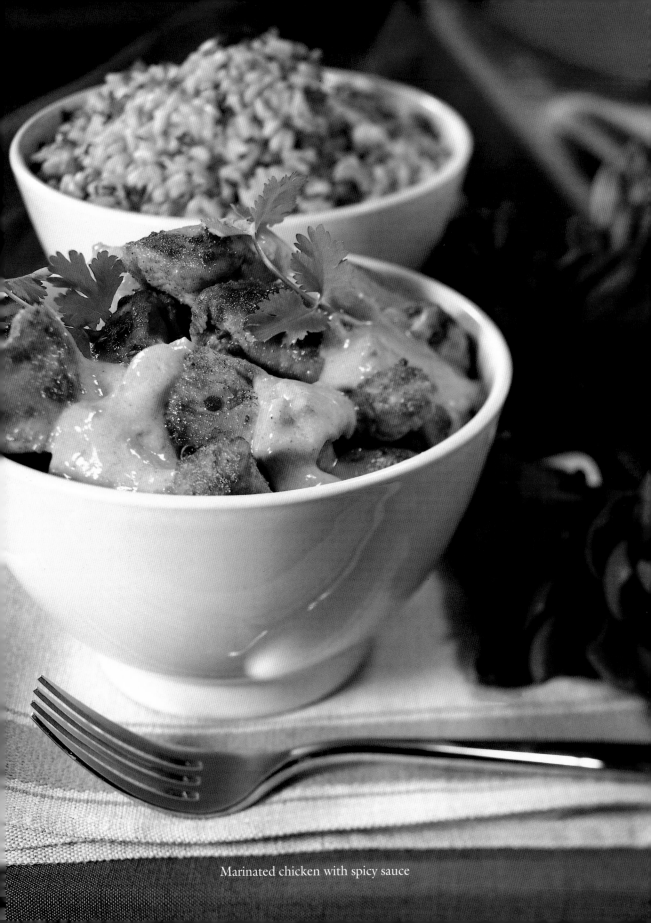

Marinated chicken with spicy sauce

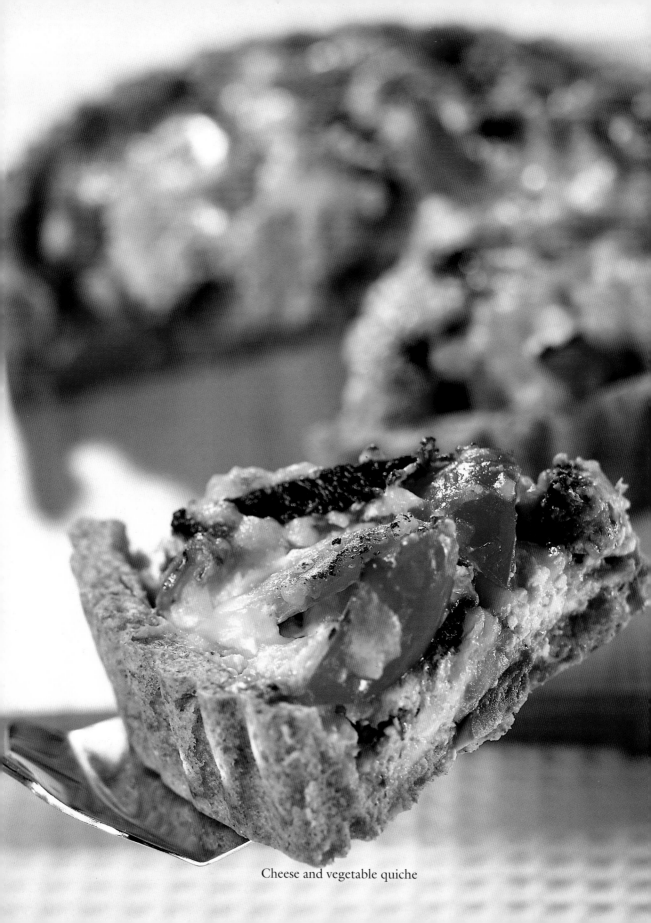

Cheese and vegetable quiche

Cheese and vegetable pizza

Ingredients   Serves 4

8oz/225g/2 cups wholemeal flour

1 teaspoon easy-bake (instant) yeast

pinch of salt

4floz/125ml/½ cup tepid water

mixed green salad to serve

 ### For the topping

4 tablespoons tomato sauce

4oz/100g/1 cup grated soya cheese

2oz/50g/scant cup mushrooms

4oz/100g/1 packed cup green beans

1 red pepper

1 onion

8 black olives

2 teaspoons olive oil

2 teaspoons dried oregano

Method

 1 Put the flour, yeast and salt in a mixing bowl. Add just enough of the water to make a firm dough. Turn out on to a floured work surface and knead for 5–10 minutes until smooth and elastic, adding more flour if the dough becomes sticky. Cover the bowl and leave to rise in a warm place for 30 minutes or until doubled in size.

 2 Heat the oven to 220°C/425°F/gas 7. Knead the dough briefly and roll into a large round. Place on a baking sheet or pizza dish. Spread with the tomato sauce and cheese.

3 Thinly slice the mushrooms, beans, red pepper and onion; pit and halve the olives. Arrange on the pizza, drizzle with oil, and sprinkle with oregano. Bake for 30 minutes until golden and bubbling. Serve with mixed green salad.

Variation

This pizza is also good made with the same quantity of sliced tofu instead of soya cheese.

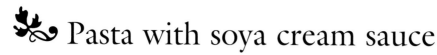 # Pasta with soya cream sauce

Ingredients Serves 4

12oz/350g/4 cups pasta shells, preferably wholewheat

salt and freshly ground black pepper

1 red pepper

1 yellow pepper

1 courgette (zucchini)

2 tablespoons sesame oil

12oz/350g/4 cups sliced button mushrooms

juice of 1 lemon

5fl oz/150ml/⅔ cup soya cream

2oz/50g/1 cup freshly grated Parmesan cheese

broccoli and tomatoes to serve

Method

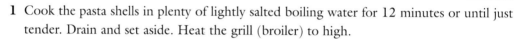

 1 Cook the pasta shells in plenty of lightly salted boiling water for 12 minutes or until just tender. Drain and set aside. Heat the grill (broiler) to high.

 2 Meanwhile core, de-seed and dice the peppers; slice the courgette (zucchini) thinly. Heat the oil in a large frying pan, add the peppers, courgette (zucchini) and mushrooms and cook for 5 five minutes, turning frequently to avoid browning.

 3 Add the pasta, lemon juice and soya cream. Stir well and season with pepper to taste.

 4 Transfer the mixture to a shallow heatproof dish, cover with the grated Parmesan cheese and grill (broil) for a few minutes until golden brown. Serve with broccoli and grilled (broiled) tomatoes.

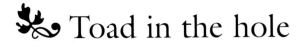 Toad in the hole

Ingredients Serves 2

4oz/100g/1 cup wholemeal flour

1 large egg

5fl oz/150ml/$\frac{2}{3}$ cup soya milk

2 tablespoons soya spread

4 soya sausages

broccoli, carrots and green beans to serve

Method

 1 Heat the oven to 220°C/425°F/gas 7. Sift the flour into a mixing bowl. Lightly beat the egg and stir into the flour, then add the milk, a little at a time to avoid lumps. Beat the mixture for 1 minute and set aside.

 2 Melt the soya spread in a flameproof dish or baking tin. Add the sausages and put in the oven for 4–5 minutes.

 3 Pour in the batter, return to the oven immediately and cook for 25 minutes until well risen.

 4 Serve with broccoli, carrots and green beans.

Sweet and sour vegetable stir-fry

Ingredients

½ red pepper

½ green pepper

4oz/100g/1 cup Chinese leaves

1 teaspoon cornflour (cornstarch)

2 tablespoons soy sauce

1 tablespoon olive oil

10oz/300g/3 cups smoked tofu

4oz/100g/1 packed cup sliced button mushrooms

10oz/300g/1¼ cups bean-sprouts

8oz/225g can pineapple chunks

freshly ground black pepper

brown rice to serve

Method

1 Core, de-seed and slice the peppers into thin strips. Shred the Chinese leaves. Mix the cornflour (cornstarch) with the soy sauce.

2 Heat the oil in a wok or large frying pan and stir-fry the peppers, Chinese leaves and tofu for 2 minutes.

3 Add the mushrooms, bean-sprouts and pineapple and continue to stir-fry for another 2 minutes.

4 Stir in the cornflour (cornstarch) mixture and cook for a further minute. Season with pepper to taste and serve with brown rice.

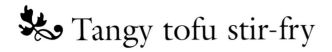 # Tangy tofu stir-fry

Ingredients Serves 4

2 x 10oz/285g packs tofu

1 red pepper

4oz/100g/1 cup button mushrooms

4 small courgettes (zucchini)

4 celery sticks

2 tablespoons sesame oil

1 pack fresh bean-sprouts

brown rice to serve

For the marinade

¾in/2cm piece fresh ginger root, grated

2 tablespoons sesame oil

2 tablespoons honey

2 tablespoons soy sauce

grated zest of 1 orange

2 teaspoons white wine vinegar

Method

1 Prepare the marinade by combining all the ingredients. Drain the tofu and slice into 1in/2.5cm cubes. Place in a shallow dish and pour the marinade over. Leave to absorb the flavours for at least 2 hours, or overnight.

2 Prepare the vegetables just before cooking: de-seed and chop the pepper, slice the mushrooms and courgettes (zucchini) and chop the celery sticks.

3 Heat the oil in a wok or large heavy frying pan. Add the bean-sprouts and all the prepared vegetables. Stir-fry for 2–3 minutes.

4 Add the tofu with its marinade and continue to stir-fry for another 2 minutes until heated through. Serve at once with brown rice.

Crunchy vegetables and pasta with smoked salmon

Ingredients   Serves 4

8oz/225g/3 cups wholewheat pasta bows

1 red onion

4 celery sticks

2 red peppers

1 green pepper

4oz/100g smoked salmon

10fl oz/300ml/1¼ cups soya cream

wholemeal bread and green salad to serve

Method

1 Bring a large pan of lightly salted water to the bowl. Add the pasta, stir once and return to the boil. Simmer for 8–12 minutes. (According to brand, and particularly with whole-wheat pasta, cooking times can vary markedly and may even be less if you like pasta firm to the bite.)

2 Meanwhile very finely dice the onion and chop the celery into ¾in/2cm pieces. De-seed the peppers and chop small. Cut the salmon into thin strips.

3 Drain the pasta and return to the pan. Add the prepared vegetables, stir in the soya cream and heat gently for 2–3 minutes.

4 Serve hot topped with strips of smoked salmon, accompanied by wholemeal bread and a green salad.

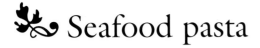 # Seafood pasta

Ingredients

8oz/225g/3 cups wholewheat pasta spirals

8oz/225g cooked peeled prawns (shrimp)

7oz/200g can crab meat or 8 crab sticks

1 red pepper

4oz/100g/1¼ cups green beans

4oz/100g/1¼ cups mangetout (snow peas)

2 tablespoons sesame oil

10oz/300g jar soya mayonnaise

2oz/50g toasted flaked almonds

Method

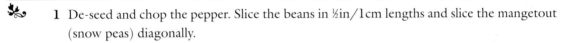

1 De-seed and chop the pepper. Slice the beans in ½in/1cm lengths and slice the mangetout (snow peas) diagonally.

2 Bring a large saucepan of lightly salted water to the boil, add the pasta, return to the boil and cook for 8–12 minutes or until done to your liking.

3 Meanwhile heat the oil in a wok or large heavy-based frying pan, add the prepared vegetables and stir-fry for 3 minutes.

4 Drain the pasta and transfer to a large warmed serving dish. Add the vegetables along with the prawns and crab meat or sliced crab sticks.

5 Stir in the soya mayonnaise, mix everything well and sprinkle with flaked almonds. Serve at once.

Smoked tofu and pasta with mixed beans

Ingredients

8oz/200g/3 cups wholewheat pasta shells

2 x 10oz/285g packs smoked tofu

8oz/225g/1¼ cups green beans

14oz/400g can mixed beans

2 tablespoons sesame oil

1 teaspoon cumin seeds

2 tablespoons virgin olive oil

freshly ground black pepper

Method

 1 Bring a large saucepan of water to the boil and cook the pasta for 8–12 minutes or until done to your liking. Drain and keep hot in a large serving dish.

 2 Meanwhile cut the tofu into cubes, slice the green beans into short lengths and drain the can of mixed beans.

 3 Heat the oil in a wok or large heavy-based frying pan. Add the cumin seeds, stir-fry for 1 minute, then add the coriander and vegetables. Stir-fry for 3 more minutes.

 4 Mix in the tofu and cook for just long enough to heat through. Transfer to the dish of pasta and mix thoroughly.

 5 Drizzle with a little virgin olive oil and season with pepper to taste. Serve at once.

Smoked tofu with bulgur wheat

Ingredients

8oz/200g/1¼ cups bulgur wheat

1 red onion

1 red pepper

10oz/300g can sweetcorn kernels

2 x 10oz/285g packs smoked tofu

3 tablespoons sesame oil

2oz/50g/½ cup sunflower seeds

Method

 1 Rinse a large heatproof bowl out with boiling water to warm it, add the bulgur wheat and pour on enough boiling water to cover. Toss with a fork and set aside.

 2 Finely chop the onion, deseed and slice the pepper and drain the sweetcorn. Cut the tofu into smallish cubes.

 3 Heat 2 tablespoons of the sesame oil in a wok or heavy-based frying pan. Stir-fry the tofu cubes until they are crisp on all sides.

 4 Add the vegetables and continue to stir-fry for a further 3 minutes.

 5 Fluff the bulgur wheat up with a fork; if necessary add a little more boiling water. The grains should have swelled and be nicely separated.

 6 Transfer the tofu and vegetable mixture to the mixing bowl and combine with the bulgur. Drizzle on the remaining oil and top with the sunflower seeds. Serve at once.

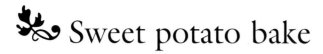 Sweet potato bake

Ingredients

1lb/500g/3 cups sweet potatoes

1lb/500g/3 cups celeriac (celery root)

1 red onion

4 green onions

4oz/100g/1 cup grated Edam cheese

1oz/25g/½ cup grated Parmesan cheese

10floz/300ml soya cream

freshly ground black pepper

1oz/25g/scant ¼ cup medium oatmeal

½oz/15g/2 tablespoons soya spread

broccoli and baked tomatoes to serve

Method

 1 Parboil the potatoes and celeriac (celery root) in separate pans. Drain and slice, cutting the celeriac (celery root) more thinly than the potatoes.

 2 Meanwhile finely chop the red onion. Trim and chop the green onions. Preheat the oven to 180°C/350°F/gas 4.

 3 Put both grated cheeses into a mixing bowl. Add the soya cream and prepared onions; mix to combine and season with pepper to taste.

 4 Grease an ovenproof dish and lay in half the potato and celeriac (celery root) slices. Spread on half the cheese mixture. Repeat the layers and sprinkle evenly with oatmeal. Dot with soya spread and bake for 1 hour until the vegetables are tender and the topping golden brown.

 5 Serve hot with broccoli and baked tomatoes.

Hazelnut and smoked tofu layer

Ingredients

8oz/225g/2 cups smoked tofu

2 tablespoons hazelnut butter

2 tablespoons soy sauce

1 clove garlic, crushed

½ teaspoon clear honey

freshly ground black pepper

stir-fried vegetables to serve

Method

1 Drain the tofu and slice it horizontally through the middle to make two thinner slices . Set aside. Heat the grill (broiler) to high.

2 Combine the hazelnut butter with the soy sauce, garlic and honey. Mix thoroughly to a paste and season with pepper to taste.

3 Spread one slice of tofu with the mixture, and place the second on top to form a sandwich. Cut the sandwich into 1in/2.5cm cubes.

4 Grill (broil) until nicely heated through and serve with stir-fried vegetables of your choice.

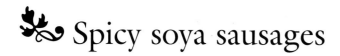 Spicy soya sausages

These sausages are equally delicious served in wholemeal pitta bread pockets, accompanied by salad; or with mashed potato, broccoli and sweetcorn. For a little luxury mix in some soya cream when mashing the potato.

Ingredients   Serves 4

8oz/225g re-hydrated soya mince

4oz/100g/2 cups wholemeal breadcrumbs

4 tablespoons soy sauce

1 small red onion

1 clove garlic, crushed

1 egg yolk

½ teaspoon ground cumin

½ teaspoon ground coriander

½ teaspoon paprika

½ teaspoon garam masala

2 tablespoons tomato paste

freshly ground black pepper

wholemeal flour for coating

Method

 1 Put the breadcrumbs and soy sauce in a mixing bowl and mix together. Chop the onion very finely and add to the bowl along with all the remaining ingredients. Mix together, using your fingers, until thoroughly combined.

 2 With moistened hands divide this mixture into 12 portions. Roll these out to form sausage shapes 4–5in/10–12cm long.

 3 Heat the grill (broiler) to high. Sprinkle some of the flour on to a plate and roll the sausages in it, trying to achieve an even coating.

 4 Grill (broil) the sausages for about 10 minutes, turning to brown all over.

Pecan nut and okra stir-fry

Ingredients Serves 4

1lb/500g/2 cups fresh okra (ladies' fingers)

1 red onion

2 cloves garlic

4oz/100g/1 cup pecan nuts

2 tablespoons sesame oil

1 tablespoon chopped fresh ginger root

3 teaspoons toasted sunflower seeds

brown rice or couscous to serve

For the miso mixture

1 tablespoon cornflour (cornstarch)

2 tablespoons water

1 tablespoon miso

1 tablespoon soy sauce

5fl oz/150ml/⅔ cup vegetable stock (bouillon)

Method

1 Prepare the miso mixture: Thoroughly mix the cornflour (cornstarch) into the water. Add the remaining ingredients and mix to produce a smooth paste.

2 Prepare the vegetables: slice the okra diagonally in 1in (2.5cm) lengths. Thinly slice the onion, crush the garlic cloves. Carefully chop the pecan nuts.

3 Heat the sesame oil in a wok or heavy-based frying pan until quite hot. Add the garlic and then the onion and grated ginger. Stir-fry for 1–2 minutes. Toss in the nuts and fry for another 3 minutes, and continue to stir, add the okra.

4 Add the miso mixture, lower the heat and cook for 3-4 more minutes. Sprinkle with the sunflower seeds and serve with brown rice or couscous.

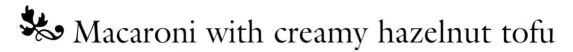# Macaroni with creamy hazelnut tofu

A mixed salad of Chinese leaf, celery, cucumber, red pepper and red onion makes the ideal accompaniment to this pasta dish. Dress the salad with homemade salad dressing (see page 36).

Ingredients   Serves 4

2 x 10oz/275g packs tofu

5fl oz/150ml/⅔ cup soya yogurt

1 tablespoon hazelnut butter

3 tablespoons yeast extract

1 tablespoon lemon juice

8oz/225g/3 cups wholewheat short-cut macaroni

freshly ground black pepper

1 tablespoon sesame seeds

mixed salad to serve

Method

  1 Put the tofu, yogurt, hazelnut butter, yeast extract and lemon juice in a blender and process until mixed and creamy.

  2 Cook the macaroni in a large saucepan of lightly salted boiling water for 8–12 minutes or until cooked to your liking. Drain, season to taste with pepper and transfer to a serving dish.

  3 Add the tofu mixture and toss together. Sprinkle the sesame seeds on top and serve at once accompanied by a mixed salad.

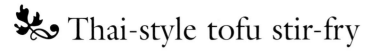 Thai-style tofu stir-fry

Ingredients Serves 4

2 x 10oz/285g packs tofu, cubed

1 red onion

3 green onions

1 red pepper

1 tablespoon sesame oil

2 tablespoons pumpkin seeds

1 tablespoon Thai green curry paste

7fl oz/200ml/1 scant cup coconut milk

6 oz/175g/1½ cups frozen petit pois, thawed

chopped fresh coriander (cilantro)

brown rice or couscous to serve

Method

1 Cut the tofu into 1in/2.5cm cubes. Finely chop the red onion; trim and shred the green onions. De-seed and finely chop the red pepper. Heat the oil in a wok or heavy-based frying pan and stir-fry the tofu for 1–2 minutes.

2 Add the curry paste, prepared red onion and the pumpkin seeds and stir-fry for 1 minute. Stir in the coconut milk, peas and red pepper and continue to cook for 5–6 minutes.

3 Transfer to a serving dish, stir in the coriander and top with the shredded onion. Serve immediately with brown rice or couscous.

❧ Citrus stir-fry

Ingredients Serves 4

2 x 10oz/285g packs tofu

1 head broccoli

4oz/100g button mushrooms

1 yellow pepper

4oz/100g/1 cup mangetout

7oz/200g can water chestnuts

7oz/200g can bamboo shoots

2 tablespoons sesame oil

❧ For the marinade

2 tablespoons sesame oil

2 tablespoons clear honey

2 tablespoons soy sauce

1 teaspoon lemon juice

2 teaspoons balsamic vinegar

1 teaspoon grated fresh ginger root

zest of 1 lime

Method

1 Cut the tofu into 1in/2.5 cm cubes. Thoroughly combine all the ingredients for the marinade and pour over the tofu.

2 Prepare the vegetables for stir-frying. Cut the broccoli into small florets and slice the mushrooms. De-seed and chop the pepper and slice the mangetout diagonally. Drain and slice the water chestnuts; drain the bamboo shoots.

3 Put the oil in a wok or large heavy-based frying pan and bring to a good heat. Toss in the broccoli florets and stir-fry for 1 minute.

4 Add all the remaining vegetables and cook for a further 2 minutes. Add the marinated tofu and continue to cook until heated through.

5 Pile the mixture on to a bed of brown rice or couscous and serve hot.

Desserts

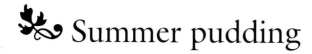 # Summer pudding

Ingredients Serves 4

1 small wholemeal loaf, thinly sliced

1½lb/700g/5 cups mixed fresh fruit (raspberries, strawberries, cherries, redcurrants, blackcurrants)

4oz/100g/¾ cup currants

2oz/50g/¼ cup sugar

½ lemon

soya cream to serve

Method

1 Lightly grease a 1½ pint/850ml/3 cup pudding bowl. Remove the crusts from the bread and arrange the slices to cover the bottom and sides of the bowl. Try to avoid gaps between the slices.

2 Prepare the fruit, halving any large strawberries. Put it all in a saucepan with the currants, sugar, grated zest and juice of the lemon and just 2 tablespoons of water.

3 Cover and bring to the boil, then simmer over a low heat for 1–2 minutes.

4 Carefully empty the contents of the pan into the bread-lined bowl without disturbing the lining, reserving 3 tablespoons of the juice.

5 Put a plate directly on top of the pudding and weight it down. Chill for about 12 hours.

6 Turn the pudding out on to a serving dish and pour the reserved juice on to any unsoaked areas. Serve with soya cream.

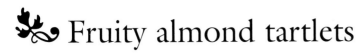 Fruity almond tartlets

Ingredients

2oz/50g/¼ cup soya spread

4oz/100g/1 cup plain (all-purpose) wholemeal flour

1oz/25g/¼ cup flaked almonds to decorate

For the filling

2oz/50g/¼ cup soya spread

1oz/25g/¼ cup soya flour

1 egg

2 tablespoons clear honey

2oz/50g/½ cup ground almonds

almond essence

3oz/75g/½ cup chopped dried apricots

Method

1 Put the soya spread in a mixing bowl with 2 tablespoons of the flour and 2 tablespoons of very cold water. Mix together with a fork. Sift in the remaining flour (return the bran to the bowl). Mix to a stiff dough, adding a little more water if necessary.

2 Flour a work surface and lightly knead the dough until smooth. Chill for 20 minutes.

3 Heat the oven to 190°C/375°F/gas 5. Make the filling: mix together the soya spread, egg, honey, ground almonds and a few drops of almond essence. Stir in the chopped apricots.

4 Roll the pastry out thinly and stamp into rounds using a 4in/10cm cutter to line 15 tartlet tins.

5 Spoon the filling into the pastry cases and sprinkle with flaked almonds. Bake for about 25 minutes until golden. Serve warm with soya cream, or eat cold.

Quick low-fat cheesecake

Traditional cheesecake is, unfortunately, as fattening as it is delicious. But this low-fat alternative clocks up very few calories, and is also very quick to make.

Ingredients   Serves 4

4 large round rice cakes
4 teaspoons low-sugar jam (jelly)
4oz/100g/½ cup soya cream cheese
fresh fruit: raspberries, strawberries, cherries, peaches
toasted flaked almonds

Method

 1 Spread each rice cake with a teaspoon of jam (jelly). Add a layer of soya cream cheese, smoothing it with a palette knife.

 2 Top each cake with fruit to taste, arranging it attractively. Raspberries can be used whole; strawberries look good if you place a circle of halved ones around a central whole berry. Halve and stone cherries and arrange them in a concentric circle; slice peaches and arrange similarly, overlapping the slices.

3 Finish by sprinkling with a few toasted flaked almonds.

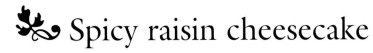 # Spicy raisin cheesecake

Ingredients Serves 8

4oz/100g/2 cups digestive biscuits (graham crackers)

2oz/50g/¼ cup soya spread

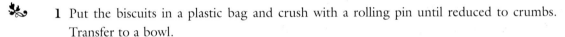

For the topping

6oz/175g/¾ cup soya cream cheese

1 egg

1 teaspoon lemon juice

2oz/50g/¼ cup caster (superfine) sugar

1 tablespoon wholemeal flour

2 tablespoons natural soya yogurt

1 teaspoon cinnamon

2oz/50g/½ cup raisins

icing (confectioners') sugar for dusting

Method

1 Put the biscuits in a plastic bag and crush with a rolling pin until reduced to crumbs. Transfer to a bowl.

2 Melt the soya spread, pour over the crumbs and mix thoroughly. Lightly oil an 8in/20cm flan tin and spread the crumb mixture evenly and firmly over the bottom.

3 Heat the oven to 170°C/325°F/gas 3. Make the topping: soften the cheese in a mixing bowl. Separate the egg and beat the yolk into the cheese. Add the lemon juice, sugar, flour, yogurt, cinnamon and raisins.

4 Whisk the egg white until stiff and fold lightly into the topping mixture. Spoon over the crumb base and level the surface with a palette knife.

5 Bake for 30 minutes or until firm but still sponge-like. Dust with icing sugar and serve warm.

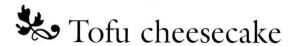 # Tofu cheesecake

Ingredients

4oz/100g/1 cup wholemeal flour

3oz/75g/6 tablespoons soya spread

3oz/75g/¾ cup ground almonds

2oz/50g caster (superfine) sugar

1 egg yolk

almond essence

For the filling

8oz/225g/2¼ cups silken tofu

5fl oz/150ml/⅔ cup natural soya yogurt

2oz/50g/¼ cup caster (superfine) sugar

1oz/25g/¼ cup cornflour (cornstarch)

3oz/75g/⅔ cup sultanas

1 lemon

2 eggs

Method

1 Put the flour in a mixing bowl, add small portions of soya spread and rub in until the mixture resembles breadcrumbs. Then stir in the ground almonds and sugar. Form a well in the centre.

2 In a separate small bowl, beat the egg yolk with 2 teaspoons of cold water and four drops of almond essence. Pour into the well in the flour mixture and stir to make a soft dough.

3 Lightly flour a work surface, turn out the dough and knead gently until smooth. Cover and chill for at least 1 hour.

4 Heat the oven to 200°C/400°F/gas 6. Roll the dough into a round large enough to line the bottom of an 8in/20cm loose-bottomed cake tin. Cover with foil and dried beans and bake for 15 minutes.

5 Remove the lining to allow the pastry to begin to brown and bake for a further 5 minutes or until golden. Take out and leave to cool. Turn down the oven to 180°C/350°F/gas 4.

6 Meanwhile make the filling. Put the tofu and yogurt in a large mixing bowl and stir together. Add the sugar, cornflour, sultanas and grated zest and juice of the lemon. Mix well.

7 Separate the eggs and stir the yolks into the mixture. Beat the whites until stiff and fold them in. Pour the cheesecake filling on to the pastry base and bake for about 30 minutes or until set and golden brown on top. Allow to cool before serving.

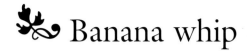 Banana whip

Ingredients

2 ripe bananas
10floz/300ml/1¼ cups soya milk
4oz/100g/½ cup cottage cheese
pinch of freshly grated nutmeg

Method

 1 Slice the bananas and put them in a blender with the soya milk.

 2 Blend for 30 seconds. Add the cottage cheese and blend for a further 30 seconds.

 3 Pour into glasses and sprinkle with nutmeg. Serve immediately.

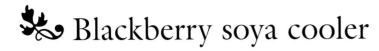 Blackberry soya cooler

Ingredients

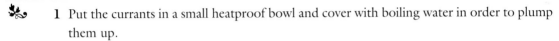
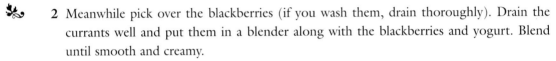

2oz/50g/½ cup currants

8oz/225g/1½ cups blackberries

15fl oz/425ml/2 cups soya yogurt

oatmeal biscuits, to serve

Method

1 Put the currants in a small heatproof bowl and cover with boiling water in order to plump them up.

2 Meanwhile pick over the blackberries (if you wash them, drain thoroughly). Drain the currants well and put them in a blender along with the blackberries and yogurt. Blend until smooth and creamy.

3 Chill before serving in tall glasses, accompanied by oatmeal biscuits.

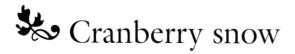 # Cranberry snow

Ingredients Serves 4

2 egg whites

10oz/300g/1¼ cups natural yogurt

2oz/50g/¼ cup caster (superfine) sugar

1lb/500g/3 cups cranberries, thawed if frozen

2 pieces stem ginger

Method

 1 Whisk the egg whites until stiff peaks are formed. Add the yogurt and use a large metal spoon to fold it gently into the egg whites; do not beat.

 2 Stir in the sugar and fold in the cranberries. Divide the mixture between four glass serving dishes.

 3 Finely chop the stem ginger and sprinkle over the top of each serving.

Variations

This dessert is equally good made with other berries such as blackberries, raspberries, blueberries or strawberries.

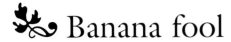 Banana fool

Ingredients Serves 4

4 ripe bananas

10oz/300g/3 cups cup silken tofu

½ teaspoon vanilla extract

1 tablespoon clear honey

2 tablespoons toasted flaked almonds

Method

 1 Chop the bananas and put into a food processor or blender. Add the tofu, vanilla extract and honey and process to a smooth purée.

 2 Spoon the mixture into four individual dishes and sprinkle with the flaked almonds.

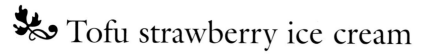# Tofu strawberry ice cream

Ingredients

1 large ripe banana

8oz/225g/1½ cups strawberries

10oz/300g/3 cups silken tofu

4 tablespoons clear honey

½ teaspoon vanilla extract

fresh mint leaves to garnish

extra fresh fruit to serve

Method

 1 Chop the banana and put the pieces on a large plate with the strawberries, in a single layer. Freeze until required.

 2 Put the frozen fruit in a food processor or blender with the tofu, honey and vanilla extract. Blend to a smooth purée, to achieve a thick creamy ice cream.

 3 Spoon into four individual dishes, or layer with extra fresh fruit and garnish with mint leaves.

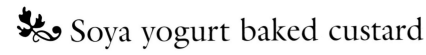 # Soya yogurt baked custard

Ingredients

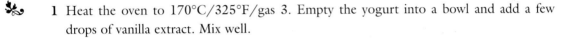
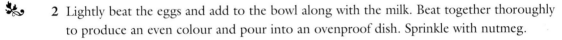

10oz/300g/1¼ cups natural soya yogurt

vanilla extract

2 eggs

5fl oz/150ml/⅔ cup soya milk

¼ teaspoon freshly grated nutmeg

Sunflower seeds or toasted flaked almonds for topping

Method

1 Heat the oven to 170°C/325°F/gas 3. Empty the yogurt into a bowl and add a few drops of vanilla extract. Mix well.

2 Lightly beat the eggs and add to the bowl along with the milk. Beat together thoroughly to produce an even colour and pour into an ovenproof dish. Sprinkle with nutmeg.

3 Place the dish on a roasting tin and surround with water to a depth of roughly 1in/2.5cm. Bake for 40 minutes or until just set firm.

4 Serve hot or cold, generously sprinkled with sunflower seeds or flaked almonds.

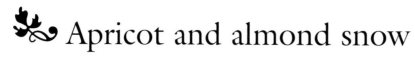 Apricot and almond snow

Ingredients Serves 4

8oz/225g/scant cup chopped dried apricots

2oz/50g/½ cup ground almonds

1 tablespoon soft brown sugar

¼ teaspoon ground cinnamon

5fl oz/150ml/⅔ cup soya yogurt

zest of 1 lemon

2 egg whites

oatmeal biscuits to serve

Method

 1 Chop the apricots until they are in very small pieces. Put in a bowl and mix with the ground almonds, sugar, cinnamon, yogurt and grated lemon zest.

 2 Whisk the egg whites until standing in stiff peaks and gently fold into the apricot mixture.

 3 Divide between four individual dishes and chill before serving accompanied by crisp oatmeal biscuits.

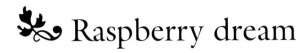 # Raspberry dream

Ingredients

2oz/50g/1 cup fresh wholemeal breadcrumbs

3oz/75g/1 cup oat cakes

1 packet blackcurrant jelly (jello)

7oz/200g/scant cup soya yogurt

6oz/175g/1½ cups raspberries, thawed if frozen

2 tablespoons flaked almonds

soya cream to serve (optional)

Method

1 Toast the breadcrumbs lightly and break up the oat cakes.

2 Mix half the breadcrumbs with all the oat cake and place in a large glass dish.

3 Make up half the jelly (jello) with hot water, according to packet instructions, and pour on to the crumbs. Put in the refrigerator until completely set.

4 Make up the remaining jelly with 6 tablespoons of hot water and chill until almost set. Whisk until frothy and stir in 2oz/50g/¼ cup of the yogurt.

5 Mix three-quarters of the raspberries into the yogurt jelly and spoon over the crumb base. Chill until set.

6 Spread the remaining yogurt over the top and sprinkle with the remaining breadcrumbs. Chill well.

7 Decorate with the remaining raspberries and sprinkle with the flaked almonds. Accompany with soya cream, served separately, if liked.

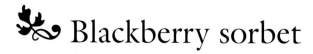 # Blackberry sorbet

Ingredients

3oz/75g/scant ½ cup sugar
1lb/500g/3 cups blackberries, thawed if frozen
grated zest and juice of ½ lemon

Method

 1 First make a sugar syrup. Put 10 fl oz/300ml/1¼ cups of water into a saucepan and add the sugar. Heat gently until the sugar has dissolved, then raise the heat and boil rapidly for 5 minutes, until syrupy. Remove from the heat and allow to cool.

 2 Sieve the blackberries into the syrup and add the lemon juice and zest. Pour into a freezer-proof bowl and freeze until firm.

 3 Remove the sorbet from the freezer 30 minutes before serving and whisk by hand until light and fluffy. Return to the refrigerator.

 4 Divide the sorbet between individual glass dishes and serve immediately.

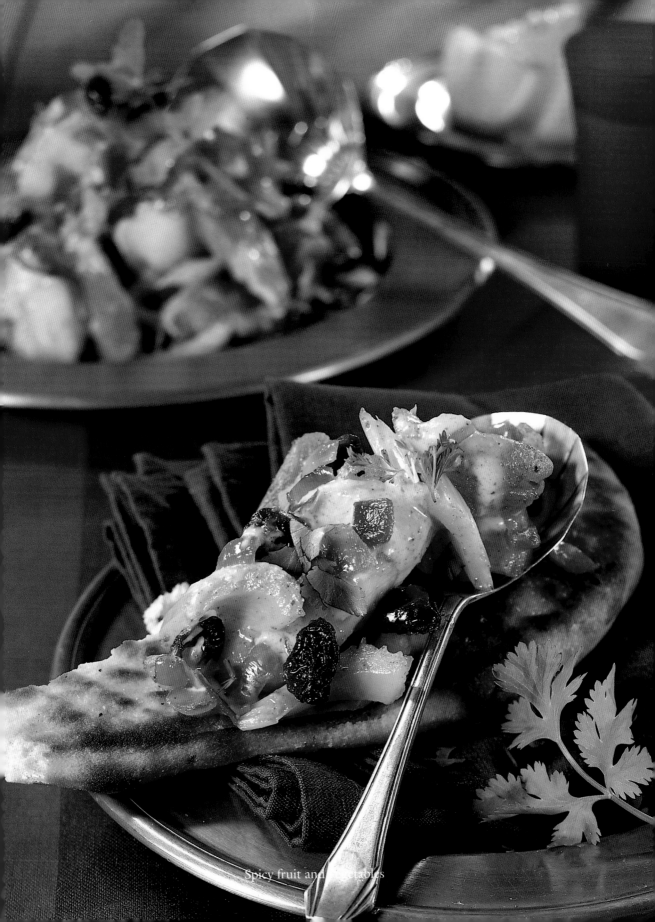

Spicy fruit and vegetables

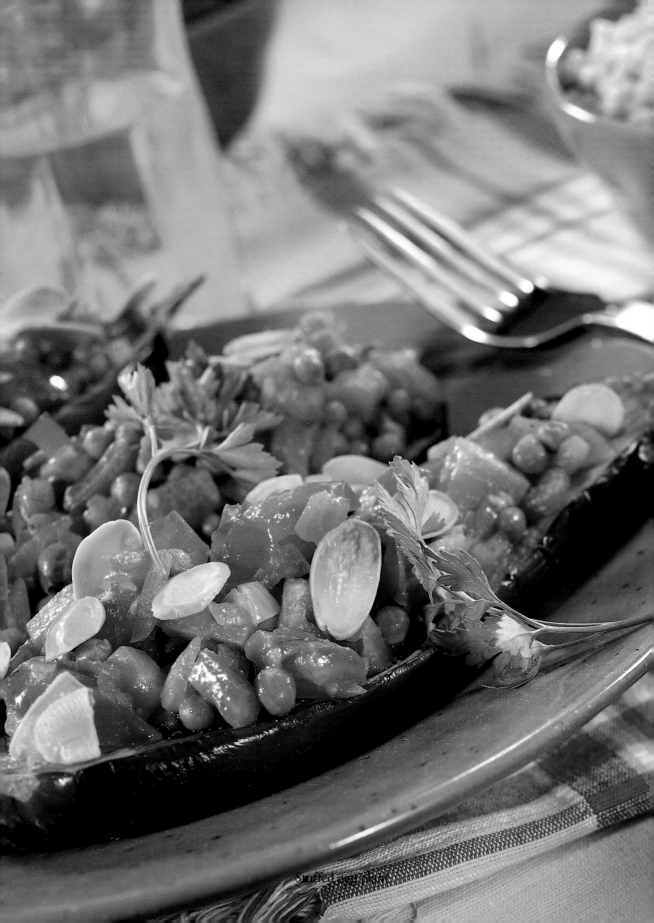

Stuffed aubergine

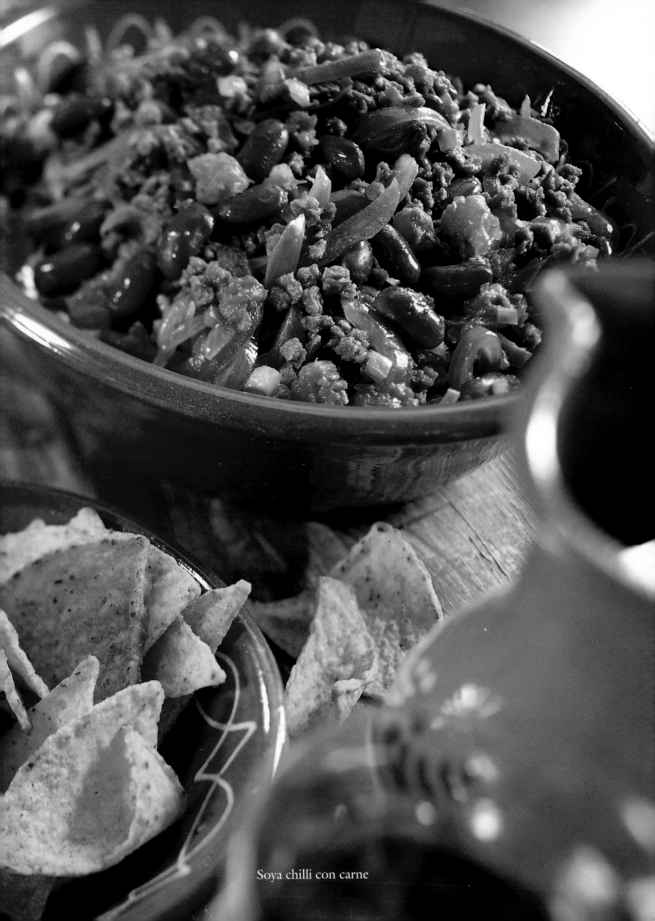

Soya chilli con carne

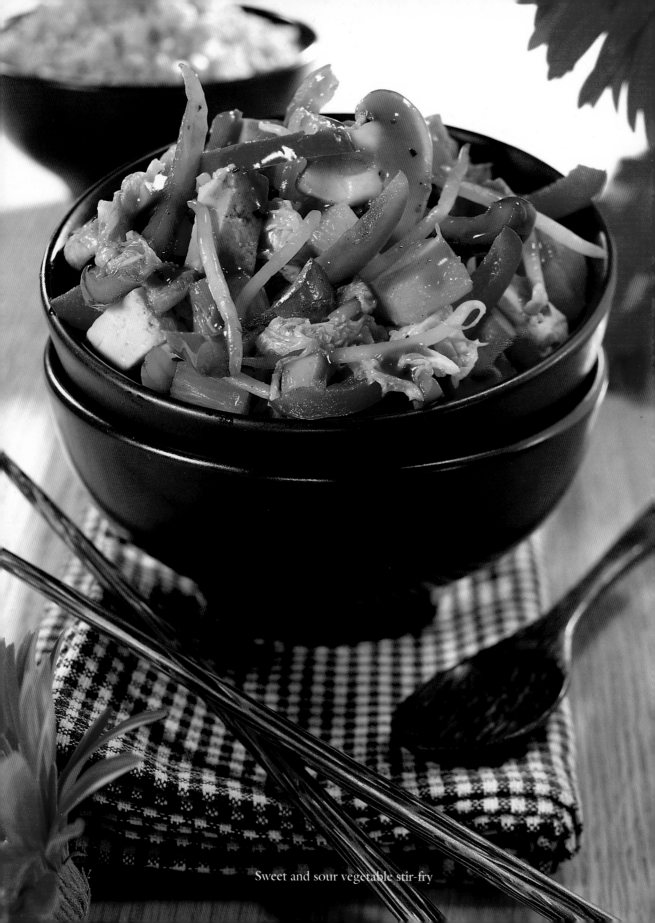

Sweet and sour vegetable stir-fry

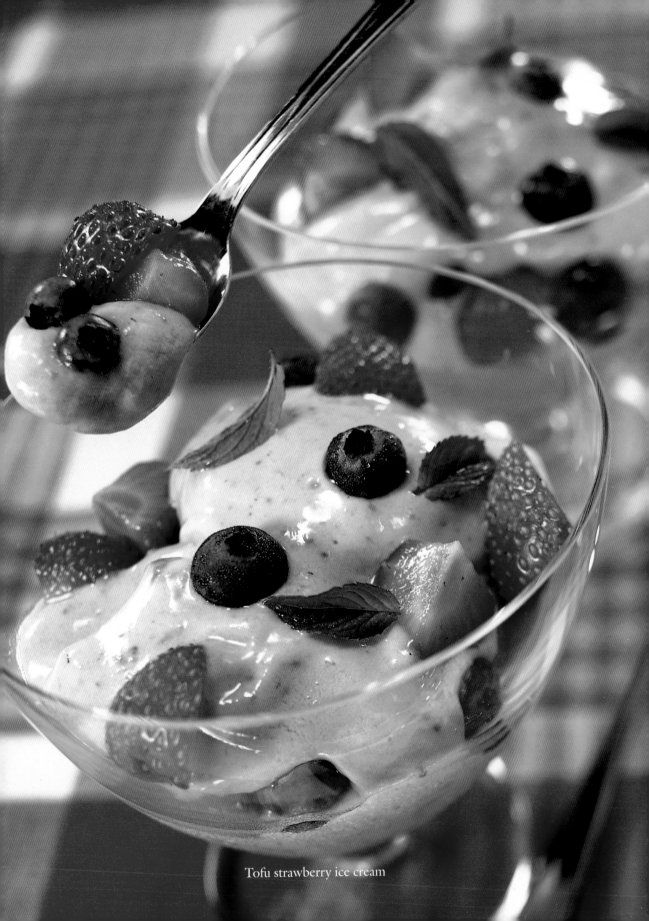

Tofu strawberry ice cream

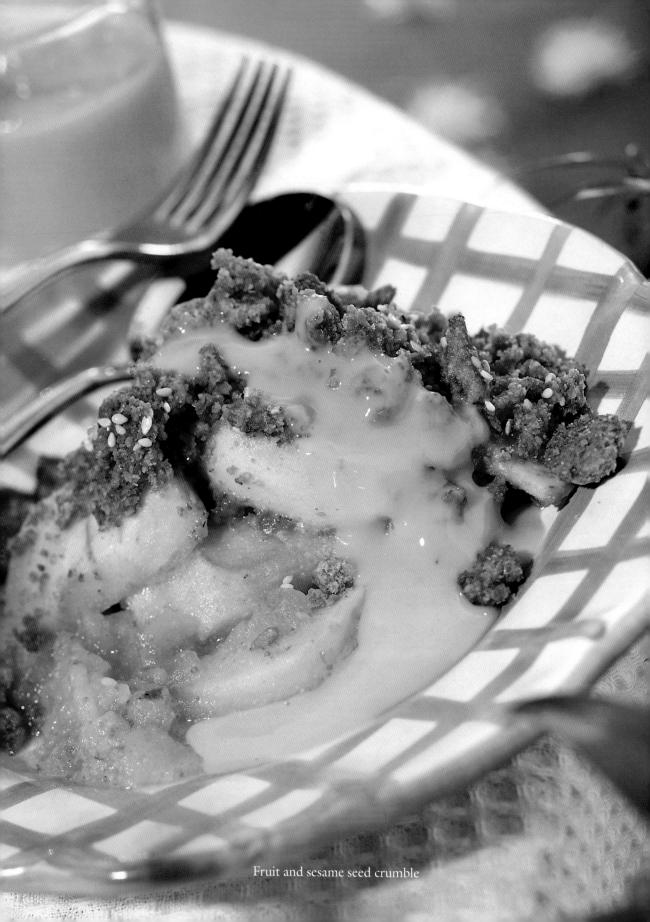

Fruit and sesame seed crumble

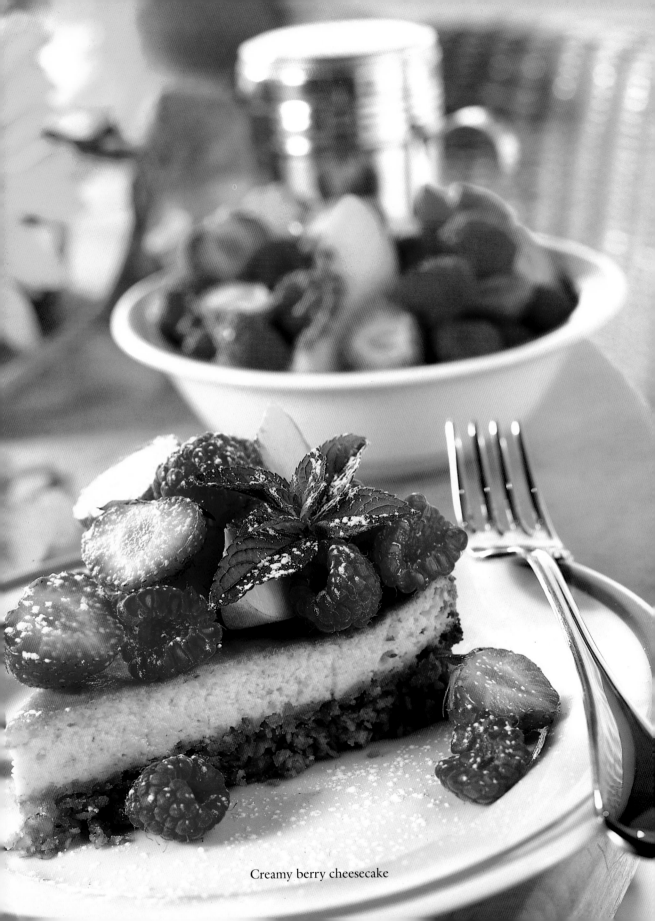

Creamy berry cheesecake

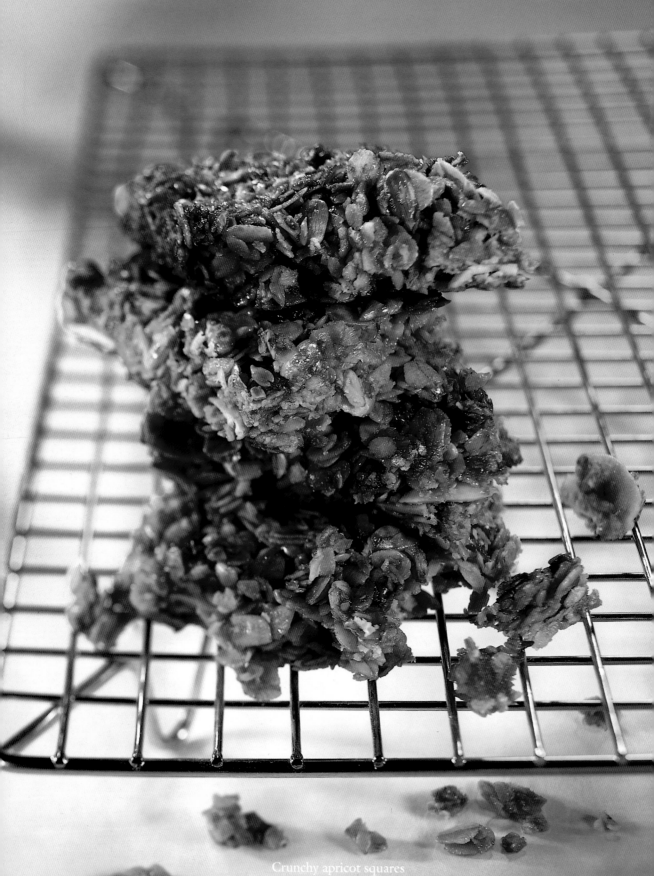
Crunchy apricot squares

Cranberry and raisin crumble

Ingredients Serves 4

8oz/225g/1½ cups cranberries

5oz/150g/1 cup raisins

4oz/100g/½ cup soft brown sugar

1 tablespoon soya flour

vanilla soya dessert to serve

 For the topping

4oz/100g/1 cup wholemeal flour

2oz/50g/¼ cup almond butter

2 oz/50g/¼ cup soft brown sugar

Method

 1 Heat the oven to 180°C/350°F/gas 4. Mix the cranberries with the raisins, sugar and flour and place in an ovenproof dish.

 2 To make the topping, first put the flour in a bowl and rub in the almond butter until the mixture resembles breadcrumbs. Stir in the sugar.

 3 Sprinkle the crumble topping over the fruit filling and bake for 30 minutes until golden and crisp. Serve with vanilla soya dessert if liked.

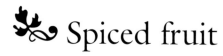 Spiced fruit

Ingredients Serves 4

4oz/100g/¾ cup dried apple slices

4oz/100g/½ cup dried apricots

4oz/100g/¾ cup dried figs

4oz/100g/1 cup dried prunes

4oz/100g/¾ cup raisins

2 cloves

1 cinnamon stick

10fl oz/300ml/1¼ cups orange juice

10fl oz/300ml/1¼ cups water

2oz/50g/½ cup toasted flaked almonds

soya cream to serve

Method

 1 Put the fruit and spices into a saucepan and pour in the orange juice and water.

 2 Cook over a moderate heat until boiling, then reduce the heat and simmer for about 20 minutes until the fruit is tender. Add more water to maintain a syrupy consistency if necessary.

 3 Pour into a serving dish and sprinkle with the toasted flaked almonds. Serve with soya cream.

Fruit and sesame seed crumble

Ingredients

1lb/500g/4 cups cooking apples

clear honey

4oz/100g/1 cup wholemeal flour

2oz/50g/¼ cup almond butter or tahini

2oz/50g/¼ cup demerara (raw) sugar

1 tablespoon sesame seeds

soya cream to serve

Method

 1 Heat the oven to 180°C/350°F/gas 4 and lightly grease a pie dish.

 2 Slice the apples thinly and put in the dish. Add honey to taste.

 3 For the topping, place the flour in a bowl and rub in the almond butter or tahini. Mix in the sugar and sprinkle the mixture over the apples.

 4 Bake for about 30 minutes until golden brown, then sprinkle with the sesame seeds and bake for a further 5 minutes. Serve hot with soya cream.

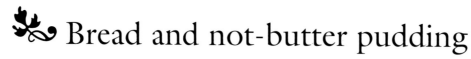 Bread and not-butter pudding

Ingredients Serves 4

6 slices wholemeal bread

soya spread

2oz/50g/½ cup raisins

2oz/50g/¼ cup soft brown sugar

3 eggs

1 pint/600ml/2½ cups soya milk

soya cream to serve

Method

  1 Cut the bread into triangles and cover with soya spread. Grease a pie dish and place half the triangles around the sides and bottom. Sprinkle the raisins over the bread with half of the sugar. Top with the remaining bread triangles.

  2 Beat the eggs and soya milk together and pour over the bread. Leave to soak for 30 minutes.

  3 Heat the oven to 180°C/350°F/gas 4. Sprinkle the remaining sugar over the top of the pudding and bake for 30–45 minutes until crisp and golden brown. Serve hot with soya cream.

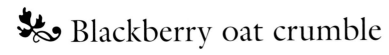 # Blackberry oat crumble

Ingredients

8oz/225g/1½ cups blackberries

1–2 tablespoons caster (superfine) sugar

Juice of 1 orange

For the topping

4oz/100g/1¼ cups rolled oats

2oz/50g/¼ cup soya spread

2oz/50g/¼ cup soft brown sugar

grated zest of 1 orange

Method

1 Heat the oven to 200°C/400°F/gas 6. Place the blackberries in a 1½/pint/850ml/4 cup pie dish. Sprinkle with the sugar and orange juice.

2 To make the topping, put the rolled oats in a bowl and rub in the soya spread. Stir in the brown sugar and orange zest. Spoon the mixture carefully over the blackberries so as to cover them completely.

3 Bake for 30 minutes until the topping is crisp and golden brown.

Apple and ginger brown Betty

Ingredients   Serves 4

3oz/75g/¾ cup soya spread

8oz/255g/2 cups muesli (granola)

1 teaspoon ground ginger

4oz/100g/½ cup raw sugar

1½lb/700g/6 cups cooking apples

1½ tablespoons sunflower seeds

1½ tablespoons flaked almonds

soya cream to serve

Method

1 Heat the oven to 180°C/350°F/gas 4. Melt the soya spread in a large saucepan and add the muesli, ginger and sugar.

2 Slice the apples thinly. Layer them in an ovenproof dish with the muesli mixture, ending with muesli to make a topping. Level and press down firmly.

3 Bake for 45 minutes until the fruit is soft and the topping crisp and golden brown. Serve hot with soya cream.

Apple and raisin dessert

       Serves 4

1 pint/600ml/2½ cups thick apple purée

4oz/100g/scant cup raisins

½ teaspoon nutmeg

juice of 1 lemon

3 teaspoons gelatine

toasted flaked almonds, for sprinkling

soya yogurt or soya ice cream to serve

Method

 1 Put the apple purée, raisins and nutmeg into a saucepan. Use the lemon juice to soften the gelatine and stir into the mixture until dissolved.

 2 Rinse a 1 pint/600ml/2 cup mould out with cold water. Spoon in the apple mixture and put in the refrigerator to set.

 3 Turn out and sprinkle with toasted flaked almonds. Serve with soya yogurt or soya ice cream.

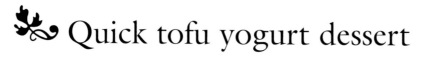 # Quick tofu yogurt dessert

Ingredients

5oz/150g/1½ cups silken tofu

5oz/150g/⅔ cup Greek (strained plain) yogurt

½ teaspoon lemon juice

2 tablespoons soft brown sugar

½ teaspoon ground cinnamon

2 round pieces of stem ginger

ratafia or pompadour biscuits to serve

Method

 1 Mix together the tofu, yogurt, lemon juice and cinnamon. Cut the stem ginger into small neat pieces and add to the mixture.

 2 Spoon the mixture into two individual dishes and cover with an even layer of soft brown sugar.

 3 Refrigerate and serve chilled with biscuits.

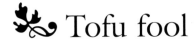 Tofu fool

Ingredients

10oz/300g/3 cups silken tofu

1 ripe banana, chopped

2 tablespoons soya cream

1 tablespoon clear honey

½ teaspoon vanilla extract

ratafia or pompadour biscuits to serve

Method

 1 Put all the ingredients in a food processor or blender and process until they form a smooth purée. Pour into a bowl and chill in the refrigerator.

 2 Serve in tall individual glasses accompanied by biscuits.

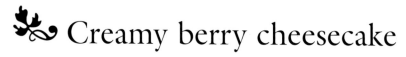 # Creamy berry cheesecake

Ingredients Serves 4-6

6oz/175g/2 cups oat cakes
3oz/75g/¾ cup soya spread
1oz/25g/⅓ cup rolled oats
2 teaspoons clear honey

For the filling

6oz/175g/¾ cup soya cream cheese
2 tablespoons soya dessert, vanilla flavour
½ teaspoon vanilla extract
1 egg, separated
1 tablespoon wholemeal flour
2oz/50g/¼ cup caster (superfine) sugar
juice of ½ lemon

For the topping

1 peach
4oz/100g/1 cup strawberries
4oz/100g/1 cup raspberries

Method

1 Heat the oven to 180°C/350°F/gas 4. Lightly oil the bottom of a 7in/18cm ring-form tin.

2 Crush the oat cakes and mix with the soya spread, oats and honey. Mould and press the mixture firmly and evenly into the bottom of the tin. Bake for 10 minutes.

3 Meanwhile make the filling. Put the soya cream cheese, vanilla dessert and essence in a bowl and mix until softened. Then add the egg yolk, flour, sugar and lemon juice and combine the whole mixture.

4 Whisk the egg white until soft peaks form, then carefully fold into the mixture. Spread the filling evenly over the crumb base and bake for 30 minutes or until the top is firm but still spongy. Leave to cool, then chill if preferred.

5 Decorate the cheesecake with the fruit just before serving, slicing the peach and halving the strawberries. Soya cream could be poured over the top as well.

Tofu raspberry ice cream

Ingredients

1 large ripe banana

8oz/225g/2 cups raspberries

10oz/300g/3 cups silken tofu

½ teaspoon vanilla extract

3 tablespoons clear honey

fresh mint leaves to garnish

extra fresh fruit to serve

Method

1 Chop the banana and lay the pieces on a plate with the raspberries in a single layer. Freeze until required to make the ice cream.

2 Put the frozen fruit into a blender or food processor with the tofu, vanilla extract and honey and process to a smooth, thick consistency.

3 Divide the ice cream between four individual glasses or layer with extra fresh fruit, garnish with fresh mint leaves and serve immediately.

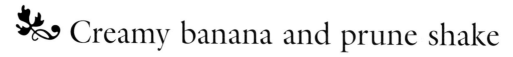 Creamy banana and prune shake

This drink is high in protein and ideal to have ready-prepared in the refrigerator for lunch times when you have no time for a proper meal.

Ingredients   Makes 2

12oz/350g/3½ cups silken tofu

1 ripe banana

10fl oz/300ml/1¼ cups unsweetened apple juice

6 pitted prunes

Method

 1 Drain the tofu and chop the banana. Put in a food processor or blender with the apple juice and prunes and process to a smooth consistency.

 2 Pour into a jug (pitcher) and chill until needed.

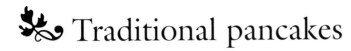 # Traditional pancakes

To give these pancakes a particular style and flavour, sprinkle the griddle or frying pan with sunflower or sesame seeds while heating it up.

Ingredients   Makes 18

4oz/100g/1 cup wheatgerm

1lb/500g/4 cups wholemeal flour

2 teaspoons baking powder

1 tablespoon brown sugar

1 teaspoon salt

2 large eggs

1½ pints/850ml/3¾ cups soya milk

2 tablespoons sunflower oil

lemon juice and caster (superfine) sugar to serve

Method

1 Sift the dry ingredients into a mixing bowl, returning the bran left behind in the sieve. Stir lightly together with a fork.

2 Lightly beat the eggs and combine with the soya milk. Stir into the dry ingredients, mixing thoroughly. Only use enough of the liquid to make a thin but creamy batter – if it is too thin the pancakes will stick; too thick and they will be heavy. Finally stir in the oil.

3 To make the pancakes use a griddle or large frying pan, un-oiled. Heat it well before pouring in a large spoonful of the batter. Cook on a medium heat for 1–2 minutes, until the surface bubbles and the edges are dryish.

4 Toss the pancake or turn with a fish slice and cook for a further minute to brown the underside.

5 Transfer the pancake to a warm plate and keep hot while you continue cooking the remainder. Serve sprinkled with sugar and lemon juice.

❧ Buckwheat pancakes

Buckwheat flour has a very strong flavour, so here I have combined it with an equal quantity of wholemeal flour. Although uncommon in the UK, buckwheat is very popular in the USA where it is used for making breakfast pancakes and muffins.

Ingredients   Makes 18 x 4in/10cm pancakes

8oz/225g/2 cups buckwheat flour

8oz/225g/2 cups wholemeal flour

½ teaspoon salt

1 tablespoon brown sugar

2 teaspoons baking powder

2 eggs

15 fl oz/450ml/2 cups soya milk

1 tablespoon sesame oil

vegetable oil for frying

soya spread and maple syrup to serve

Method

❧ 1 Sift the flours into a mixing bowl, returning any bran left behind in the sieve. Add the salt, sugar and baking power and stir them in lightly.

❧ 2 Beat the eggs and add to the bowl with the milk and oil. Stir just enough to mix the ingredients together.

❧ 3 Lightly oil a hot griddle or large frying pan and cook spoonfuls of the batter in the same way as for traditional pancakes. Due to the relatively heavy nature of the main ingredients they take rather longer to cook. The appearance of bubbles on the surface shows they are ready for turning.

❧ 4 Serve hot with soya spread and maple syrup.

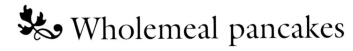# Wholemeal pancakes

Ingredients

2oz/50g/½ cup wholemeal flour

½ teaspoon baking powder

5fl oz/150ml/⅔ cup soya milk

1 egg white

vegetable oil for frying

honey and soya cream to serve

Method

1 Sift the flour and baking powder into a bowl (return the bran to the bowl) and gradually whisk in the milk. Whisk the egg white until stiff and fold into the batter.

2 Brush a non-stick frying pan with oil and heat gently. Pour in a quarter of the batter and tilt the pan to coat it evenly. Cook the pancake for 1–2 minutes until the underside is brown, then turn over for a few seconds.

3 Continue in this way, removing the pancakes as they are cooked and stacking them between lightly oiled foil. Keep hot. Serve with honey and soya cream.

Cakes, cookies and sweet snacks

Linda's 'Beat the menopause' cake

This cake is 95% fat free – no fat is added as this is provided by the nuts and seeds.

Ingredients
Makes 7 slices

4oz/100g/1 cup soya flour

4oz/100g/1 cup wholemeal flour

4oz/100g/1 scant cup rolled oats

4oz/100g/½ cup linseeds

2oz/50g/½ cup sunflower seeds

2oz/50g/½ cup pumpkin seeds

2oz/50g/½ cup sesame seeds

2oz/50g/½ cup flaked almonds

2 pieces stem ginger, finely chopped

8oz/225g/1½ cups raisins

½ teaspoon nutmeg

½ teaspoon cinnamon

½ teaspoon ground ginger

about 15fl/oz/425ml/2 cups soya milk

1 tablespoon malt extract

Method

 1 Put all the dry ingredients into a large mixing bowl. Add the soya milk and malt extract, mix well and leave to soak for about 30 minutes.

 2 Heat the oven to 190°C/375°F/gas 5. Line a small loaf tin with baking parchment.

 3 If the mixture ends up too stiff – it should have a soft dropping consistency, just too thick to pour – stir in some more soya milk. Spoon the mixture into the prepared tin and bake for 1¼ hours. Test with a skewer and if it is not cooked through allow 5–10 more minutes.

4 Turn out and cool on a wire rack. Eat in thick slices with soya spread.

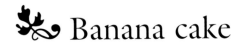 # Banana cake

Ingredients

Makes one 7in/18cm cake

2 ripe bananas

4oz/100g/½ cup soya spread

4 tablespoons clear honey

2 eggs

4oz/100g/1 cup plain (all-purpose) wholemeal flour

2 teaspoons baking powder

For the filling

1 small banana

1 teaspoon lemon juice

2oz/50g/¼ cup natural soya cream cheese

2 tablespoons ground almonds

1 teaspoon clear honey

Method

1 Line two 7in/18cm sandwich tins (layer cake pans) with baking parchment. Heat the oven to 180°C/350°F/gas 4.

2 Put the two ripe bananas in a mixing bowl and mash thoroughly. Mix in the honey and soya spread with a fork, then add the eggs. Sift in the flour (return the bran to the bowl) and baking powder. Beat thoroughly together until smooth.

3 Divide the mixture between the prepared tins and bake for 20–25 minutes. The cakes should be spongy to the touch. Leave to cool on a wire rack.

4 Meanwhile mix all the filling ingredients together until smooth and creamy. Sandwich the filling between the two cakes. Eat within 2 days.

CAKES, COOKIES AND SWEET SNACKS 127

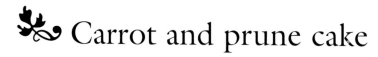 Carrot and prune cake

Ingredients

Makes 16 slices

4oz/100g/²/₃ cup carrots

4oz/100g/¹/₂ cup prunes

2oz/50g/¹/₄ cup soya spread

6 tablespoons clear honey

3oz/75g/1 cup ground almonds

¹/₄ teaspoon sunflower oil

8oz/225g/2 cups brown rice flour

1 teaspoon bicarbonate of soda (baking soda)

¹/₂ teaspoon cream of tartar

¹/₂ teaspoon ground cinnamon

1 egg

4 fl oz/125ml/¹/₂ cup soya milk

3 tablespoons unsweetened apple juice

Method

 1 Line a 6in/15cm square cake tin with baking parchment. Heat the oven to 180°C/ 350°F/gas 4.

 2 Grate the carrots; stone and chop the prunes.

 3 Melt the soya spread and honey in a small saucepan. Put the ground almonds, sunflower oil, flour, bicarbonate (baking soda), cream of tartar and cinnamon in a mixing bowl and stir together.

 4 Beat the egg, soya milk and apple juice together until combined and add to the bowl. Add the soya spread and honey mixture and stir until all the ingredients are thoroughly mixed.

 5 Pour into the prepared tin and bake for 1 hour. Cool on a wire rack.

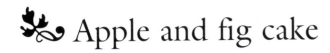 Apple and fig cake

Ingredients

8oz/225g/2 cups plain (all-purpose) wholemeal flour

2 teaspoons baking powder

2 teaspoons ground mixed (pie) spice

3 tablespoons clear honey

8oz/225g/1½ cup dried chopped figs

4fl oz/125ml/½ cup apple juice

4fl oz/125ml/½ cup sunflower oil

2 eating apples

2 tablespoons sunflower seeds

Greek (strained plain) yogurt or soya cream to serve

Method

1 Grease and line an 8in/20cm round deep cake tin. Heat the oven to 180°C/350°/gas 4.

2 Sift the flour into a mixing bowl, returning the bran, and add the baking powder and mixed (pie) spice. Make a well in the centre and add the honey, chopped figs, apple juice and sunflower oil.

3 Core and grate the apples into the bowl. Beat until thoroughly mixed, then turn into the prepared tin and sprinkle with the sunflower seeds.

4 Bake for 1–1¼ hours until the cake springs back when pressed in the centre. Turn out on to a wire rack to cool. Serve with Greek (strained plain) yogurt or soya cream.

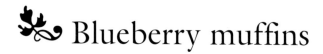 # Blueberry muffins

Ingredients

9oz/250g/2¼ cups plain (all-purpose) flour

1 tablespoon baking powder

3oz/75g/scant ½ cup caster (superfine) sugar

2 oz/50g/½ cup ground almonds

4oz/100g/½ cup soya spread

3 eggs

8fl oz/250ml/1 cup soya milk

vanilla extract

6oz/175g/1 packed cup blueberries

2 tablespoons soft brown sugar

2oz/50g/½ cup flaked almonds

strawberries or raspberries and soya cream to serve (optional)

Method

1 Heat the oven to 200°C/400°F/gas 6. Line a 12-cup muffin tin with paper cases.

2 Sift the flour into a large mixing bowl, add the baking power, caster sugar and ground almonds and stir together.

3 Melt the soya spread. Lightly beat the eggs and whisk in the soya spread with the milk. Add a few drops of vanilla extract, then fold into the flour mixture. It should remain fairly lumpy. Stir in the blueberries until evenly mixed.

4 Spoon the mixture into the paper cases. Top each muffin with brown sugar and flaked almonds and bake for 25–30 minutes until well risen and golden.

5 Remove from the tin while still warm and cool on a wire rack. For a special treat serve with soft fruit and soya cream.

Apple and currant muffins

Ingredients

8oz/225g/2 cups plain (all-purpose) wholemeal flour

pinch of salt

1 tablespoon baking powder

2oz/50g/¼ cup caster (superfine) sugar

2oz/50g/¼ cup soya spread

2 eggs

5fl oz/150ml/⅔ cup soya milk

1 eating apple

2oz/50g/½ cup currants

Method

1 Heat the oven to 220°C/425°F/gas 7. Grease two bun tins (or use paper cases).

2 Sift the flour into a mixing bowl, putting the bran remaining in the sieve back into the bowl. Stir in the salt, baking power and sugar.

3 Melt the soya spread. Beat the eggs and add the soya milk and melted spread. Rapidly stir this liquid into the flour mixture, without beating – speed is important.

4 Grate the apple into the mixture and fold in with the currants.

5 Spoon into the bun tins or paper cases so they are about one-third full. Bake for 20 minutes and serve hot.

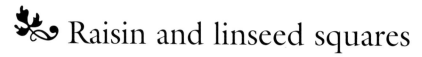 Raisin and linseed squares

Ingredients

3 tablespoons malt extract

2 tablespoons clear honey

4fl oz/125ml/½ cup sunflower oil

4oz/100g/1 cup jumbo oats

4oz/100g/1¼ cups rolled oats

1oz/25g/¼ cup sunflower seeds

1oz/25g/¼ cup linseeds

4oz/100g/¾ cup raisins

Method

  1 Heat the oven to 180°C/350°F/gas 4. Grease a 12 × 8in/30 × 20cm Swiss roll tin (sheet cake pan).

  2 Place the malt extract, honey and sunflower oil in a saucepan and heat gently until combined. Remove from the heat and mix with the rest of the ingredients, stirring thoroughly.

  3 Press the mixture into the prepared tin and smooth the top with a spatula. Bake for 30 minutes.

  4 Cool in the tin for 5 minutes, then cut into squares. Store in an airtight tin.

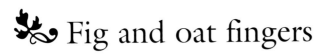# Fig and oat fingers

Ingredients

8oz/225g/1½ cups dried chopped figs

3 tablespoons apple juice

6fl oz/175/ml/¾ cup sunflower oil

4 tablespoons clear honey

6oz/175g/1½ cups plain (all-purpose) wholemeal flour

6oz/175g/2 cups rolled oats

2oz/50/½ cup chopped walnuts

½ teaspoon ground cinnamon

1 tablespoon linseed

Method

1 Grease and line an 8in/20cm square shallow cake tin. Heat the oven to 190°C/375°F gas 5.

2 Put the figs and apple juice into a small saucepan and simmer for 5 minutes until soft.

3 Pour the oil and honey into a larger saucepan and heat gently until evenly blended. Stir in the flour, oats, walnuts, cinnamon and linseed and mix together thoroughly.

4 Turn half the mixture out into the cake tin, spreading evenly and firmly. Cover with the figs and top with the remaining oat mixture.

5 Bake for 30–35 minutes or until golden brown. Allow to cool for a few minutes before cutting into fingers. Remove from the tin when cold.

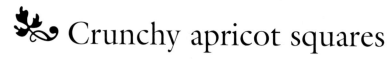 # Crunchy apricot squares

Ingredients

3 tablespoons malt extract

2 tablespoons clear honey

4 fl oz/100ml/½ cup sunflower oil

4oz/100g/1 cup jumbo oats

1oz/25g/¼ cup linseed

1oz/25g/¼ cup sunflower seeds

1oz/25g/¼ cup flaked almonds

4oz/100g/½ cup finely chopped dried apricots

4oz/100g/1¼ cups rolled oats

Method

 1 Heat the oven to 180°C/350°F/gas 4. Grease a 12 × 8in/30 × 20cm Swiss roll tin (sheet cake pan).

 2 Put the malt extract, honey and oil in saucepan and heat gently until combined. Remove from the heat and add all the remaining ingredients. Stir together thoroughly.

 3 Put the mixture in the prepared tin and level the top with a spatula. Bake for 30 minutes or until golden. Leave to cool in the tin for a few minutes, then mark off into squares. Remove from the tin when completely cool.

Linseed and sunflower snaps

Ingredients

5oz/150g/1½ scant cups rolled oats

1oz/25g/¼ cup linseed

1oz/25g/¼ cup sunflower seeds

1 tablespoon sesame seeds

1 egg

4 tablespoons clear honey

4fl oz/125ml/½ cup sunflower oil

Method

1 Heat the oven to 180°C/350°F/gas 4. Put all the dry ingredients in a mixing bowl. Lightly beat the egg and add to the bowl along with the honey and sunflower oil. Stir together thoroughly.

2 Drop teaspoonfuls of the mixture on to a baking sheet, spacing them well apart. Flatten each one with a moistened spatula.

3 Bake for 15 minutes until golden brown. Leave for a few minutes before transferring to a wire rack to finish cooling.

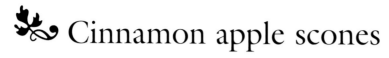# Cinnamon apple scones

Ingredients

Makes about 12

4oz/100g/1 cup plain (all-purpose) wholemeal flour

4oz/100g/1 cup soya flour

½ teaspoon bicarbonate of soda (baking soda)

1 teaspoon cream of tartar

1 teaspoon ground cinnamon

1 eating apple

2oz/50g/¼ cup soya spread

6 tablespoons soya milk

1 tablespoon clear honey

sesame seeds and soya milk for glazing

Method

1 Heat the oven to 220°C/425°F/gas 7. Dust a baking sheet with flour.

2 Sift the dry ingredients into a mixing bowl, returning the bran left behind from the flour to the bowl.

3 Grate the apple and add to the bowl along with the soya spread, milk and honey. Mix together with a fork to produce a soft dough.

4 Flour a work surface generously and knead the dough lightly. Roll out to a thickness of ¾in/2cm.

5 Using a 2in/5cm cutter (plain or fluted, as preferred) stamp the dough into rounds.

6 Place on the baking sheet, brush with soya milk and sprinkle with sesame seeds. Bake for about 15 minutes, then place on a wire rack to cool.

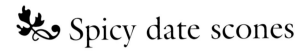 Spicy date scones

Ingredients

4oz/100g/1 cup plain (all-purpose) flour

4oz/100g/1 cup plain (all-purpose) wholemeal flour

2 tablespoons caster (superfine) sugar

½ teaspoon bicarbonate of soda (baking soda)

½ teaspoon cream of tartar

1 teaspoon ground mixed (pie) spice

2oz/50g/¼ cup soya spread

2oz/50g/scant ½ cup chopped dried dates

about 4fl oz/125ml/½ cup soya milk

Method

1 Heat the oven to 190°C/375°F/gas 5. Grease and flour a baking sheet.

2 Sift the flours into a mixing bowl, returning the bran left in the sieve. Add the remaining dry ingredients and mix thoroughly, then rub in the soya spread. Add the dates and stir in just enough milk to make a firm dough.

3 Flour a work surface, turn the dough out on to it and knead lightly. Roll out to a thickness of roughly ½in/1cm and cut out ten or so rounds.

4 Lay the scones on the prepared baking sheet and brush sparingly with soya milk. Bake for about 20 minutes and cool on a wire rack.

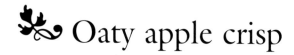 Oaty apple crisp

Ingredients

4 crisp green apples

Juice of ½ lemon

½ teaspoon cinnamon

1 tablespoon wholemeal flour

3oz/75g/⅔ cup raisins

2 tablespoons apple juice or water

 For the topping

4oz/100g/1¼ cups rolled oats

2oz/40g/½ cup toasted wheatgerm

2oz/50g/½ cup wholemeal flour

¼ teaspoon salt

1 tablespoon cinnamon

2oz/50g/¼ cup brown sugar

2oz/50g/¼ cup soya spread

Method

 1 Heat the oven to 190°C/375°F/gas 5. Slice the apples into a bowl and sprinkle with the lemon juice. Add the flour, raisins, cinnamon and the apple juice or water. Mix together.

 2 Transfer the apple mixture to a baking dish measuring about 9 × 13in/23 × 33cm. Mix the topping ingredients together in a bowl and sprinkle evenly over the top.

3 Press down well and bake for about 30 minutes. Eat hot or warm.

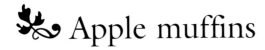 # Apple muffins

Ingredients

2oz/50g/¼ cup soya spread

2 eggs

5fl oz/150ml/⅔ cup soya milk

1 eating apple

8oz/200g/2 cups plain (all-purpose) wholemeal flour

pinch of salt

2oz/50g/¼ cup caster (superfine) sugar

Method

1 Heat the oven to 220°C/425°F/gas 7. Grease a 12-cup muffin tin.

2 Melt the soya spread. Beat the eggs in a mixing bowl and add the milk and melted soya spread. Peel and grate the apple.

3 Sift the flour, salt and sugar into a separate bowl, returning the bran left behind in the sieve. Quickly stir in the liquid mixture – speed is essential – but do not beat.

4 Fold in the grated apple and spoon the mixture into the prepared tins so they are about one-third full. Bake for 25 minutes or until well risen and golden. Serve hot.

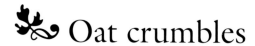 Oat crumbles

Ingredients Makes 24

2 tablespoons malt extract

2 tablespoons clear honey

2fl oz/50ml/¼ cup sunflower oil

4oz/100g/1 cup jumbo oats

4oz/100g/1¼ cups rolled oats

1oz/25g/¼ cup sunflower seeds

1oz/25g/¼ cup pumpkin seeds

1oz/25g/¼ cup linseed

2 tablespoons soya flour

4fl oz/125ml/½ cup soya milk

Method

 1 Heat the oven to 180°C/350°F/gas 4. Grease a 12 × 6in/30 × 20cm Swiss roll tin (sheet cake pan).

 2 Place the malt extract, honey and oil in a saucepan and heat gently until melted. Remove from the heat and combine with the rest of the ingredients, mixing thoroughly.

 3 Press the mixture into the prepared tin and smooth the top with a spatula. Bake for 30 minutes, then cool in the tin for 5 minutes.

 4 Cut into squares and allow to cool completely before removing from the tin.

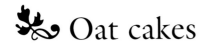 # Oat cakes

Ingredients

4oz/100g/¾ cup medium oatmeal, plus extra for kneading the dough

½ teaspoon salt

pinch of bicarbonate of soda (baking soda)

2 teaspoons soya (canola) oil

about 2fl oz/50ml/¼ cup hot water

almond butter to serve

Method

1 Put the oatmeal, salt and bicarbonate of soda (baking soda) into a bowl and mix together. Make a well in the centre, pour in the oil and enough hot water to make a stiff dough.

2 Sprinkle your hands and a board with oatmeal and knead the dough until there are no cracks in it. Flatten and roll it into a round ¼in/6mm thick.

3 Heat a griddle or heavy-based frying pan and grease lightly. Cut the round into four triangles and lift on to the cooking surface with a palette knife or fish slice.

4 Cook over a moderate heat for about 20 minutes, until the oat cakes curl up at the corners. Turn and cook on the other side for 5 minutes. Serve with almond butter.

Useful addresses

UK

Menopausal Helpline
228 Muswell Hill Broadway
London N10 3SH
Please send an SAE for information.

Women's Nutritional Advisory Service
P.O. Box 268
Lewes
East Sussex
BN7 2QN
Tel: 01273 487 366

Amarant Trust
Grant House
56–60 St John Street
London
EC1M 4DT
Tel: 0171 490 1644

Woman's Health Concern
83 Earls Court Road
London
W8 6EF
Tel: 0171 938 3932

Women's Health and Reproductive Rights
Information Centre
52 Featherstone Street
London
EC1Y 8RT
Tel: 0171 251 6580

Natural Progesterone Information Society
P.O. Box 131
Etchingham
TN19 7ZN
Contact for further information and a list of
doctors able to prescribe natural progesterone.

National Osteoporosis Society
P.O. Box 10
Radstock
Bath
BA3 3YB

The Nutri Centre
7 Park Crescent
London W1N 3HE
Tel: 0171 436 5122
Stocks wide range of nutritional supplements,
both in the shop or via mail order.

The Institute for Optimum Nutrition
Blades Court
Deodar Road
London SW15 2NU
Tel: 0181 877 9993

Soya and Health Foods:
Toffuti UK Ltd
5th Floor Congress House
14 Lyon Road
Harrow
HA1 2FD
Tel: 0181 861 4443

Allergy Care
9 Corporation Street
Taunton
Somerset
TA1 4AJ
Tel: 01823 325 023

Australia

Australian Nutrition Foundation
1–3 Derwent Street
Glebe
NSW 2037
Tel: 02 9552 3081

Women's Health Advisory Service
155 Eaglecreek Road
Werombi 2571
NSW 2570
Tel: 046 331 445

National Herbalists' Association of Australia
P.O. Box 61
Broadway
NSW 2007
Tel: 02 9211 6437

New Zealand

Health Alternative for Women
Room 101, Cranmer Ctr
P.O. Box 884
Christchurch
Tel: 03 796 970

New Zealand Nutrition Foundation
P.O. Box 33/1409
Takapuna
Auckland
Tel: 09 9486 2036

Women's Health Collective
63 Ponsonby Road
Ponsonby
Auckland
Tel: 764 506

USA

North American Menopause Society
P.O. Box 94527
Cleveland,
Ohio 44101
Tel: (440) 442 7550
www.menopause.org

American Dietetic Association
National Center for Nutrition and Dietetics
216 West Jackson Blvd., Suite 800
Chicago
Illinois 60606-6995
Tel: (800) 342 2383
www.eatright.org

Women's Health Advocate Newsletter
P.O. Box 420235
Palm Coast
Florida 32142-0235
Tel: (800) 829 5876

National Women's Health Network
1325 G Street, N.W.
Washington, DC 20005

Soya and Health Foods:
Mountain Ark Trader
P.O. Box 3170
Fayetteville
AR 72701
Tel: (800) 647 8909

Ener-g Foods Inc.
P.O. Box 84487
Seattle
WA 98124-4787
Tel: (800) 331 5222

Index